NONI JUICE

How Much, How Often, For What

THIRD EDITION

Contains information from more than 25,000 noni juice drinkers

Noni Juice: How Much, How Often, For What
Direct Source Publishing
15 East 400 South
Orem, Utah 84058

For questions or comments concerning noni use directed to the author, please send correspondence to the above address.

No information contained here is meant to replace the advice of your doctor or healthcare practitioner. The data and opinions appearing in this book are for informational purposes only. Dr. Neil Solomon does not offer medical advice, and he encourages readers to seek advice from qualified health professionals.

ISBN 1-887938-90-7

I dedicate this book to the love of my life—my dear wife, Frema, who makes me very happy. To our three special sons and their wives: Ted and Esther, Scott and Florita, and Cliff and Bernadette. And to our precious grandchildren, Scott, Jacob, Bayard, Tessa Grace, and Isabella Rose.

"I believe that ounce for ounce TAHITIAN NONI® Juice is the most potent healing food on the planet."

Dr. Samuel Kolodney

"TAHITIAN NONI® Juice is a miracle from paradise that the whole world needs to hear about."

Floyd Holdman

"TAHITIAN NONI® Juice has made a tremendous impact on my life. Many thanks to you, Dr. Solomon, for helping all of the thousands of people you haven't even met."

Denise Mata

"TAHITIAN NONI® Juice has given me the opportunity to offer my patients conventional medicine as well as a holistic approach. The results have been absolutely amazing and, at times, a miracle."

Dr. Orlando Pile, M.D.
Internist

"The fascinating story of how this ancient herbal drug can alleviate or even cure certain medical problems is a story that ideally should be told by a medical doctor who has advanced training in biochemistry and who has the writing skills to make a complicated story intelligible and interesting. Dr. Neil Solomon is this ideal person. "

Ralph Heinicke, Ph.D.
Former Director of Basic Research at Dole, Inc.

About the Author

Since the 1950s, Neil Solomon, M.D., Ph.D. has devoted his life to the study and practice of medicine. In 1961 he graduated with honors from Case-Western Reserve University in Cleveland, Ohio, with a Medical Degree (M.D.) and a Master of Science degree in Integrated Biological Sciences. Later he did his clinical training on the celebrated Osler Medical Service at the Johns Hopkins Hospital in Baltimore, Maryland. At the Johns Hopkins Medical Institution, he won the coveted Schwentker Award for excellence in research and was a member of the faculty.

While on the Johns Hopkins Medical School faculty, Dr. Solomon spent two years with the National Institutes of Health conducting research in the fields of nutrition, physiology, medicine, gerontology, endocrinology, and heart disease. It was during this time that Dr. Solomon received his doctorate in physiology, with minors in biochemistry and biophysics from the University of Maryland School of Medicine. For a decade (1969-1979), Dr. Solomon served as the first Secretary of Health and Mental Hygiene in the State of Maryland.

Dr. Solomon is retired from the practice of medicine. He is a consultant to international corporations and to NGO's of the United Nations. Dr. Solomon has also published several books, and is a New York Times best-selling author. In addition, he has enjoyed being a radio and television talk show host, the first health commentator on CNN/TV, and a medical columnist for the Los Angeles Times Syndicate for over 18 years. His interest in preventative medicine and natural healing has motivated him to write and record over a dozen other works about Morinda citrifolia besides this one.

Some of Dr. Solomon's other educational information on noni includes:

Doctor to Doctor 2nd Edition
What is Noni?
The Noni Solution
Cancer—How & Why Noni Helps
Happy & Healthy Pets
The Noni Phenomenon
The Pain Fighter: TAHITIAN NONI® Juice

These titles are available from Direct Source Publishing by calling 1-800-748-2996 or visiting www.nonitools.com.

Table of Contents

Acknowledgments i

Amazing Noni Juice 1

Noni is Safe 5

The Noni Phenomenon 7

Suggested Noni Usage 9

Section One: Cancer 15

Section Two: Arthritis 22

Section Three: Fibromyalgia and Energy 27

Section Four: Diabetes 32

Section Five: Asthma, Respiratory Problems, and Allergies 36

Section Six: Depression 39

Section Seven: Multiple Sclerosis 43

Section Eight: High Blood Pressure, Heart Disease, and Stroke . .46

Section Nine: HIV and other Immune System Disorders 49

Section Ten: Acute and Chronic Pain 54

Section Eleven: Menstrual Disorders 58

Section Twelve: Obesity 61

Section Thirteen: Kidney Disease 65

Section Fourteen: Skin and Hair Problems 68

Section Fifteen: Smoking 71

Section Sixteen: Mental Acuity
    (Memory and Concentration Difficulties) 73

Section Seventeen: Health Enhancers—Muscle Building,
    Sexual Enhancement, Better Sleep,
    Better Digestion, Well-being. 76

Question and Answer 78

Endnotes 84

Acknowledgments

As I recall the many people who in some way contributed to this book, there are simply too many to recognize in this limited space. However, I will do my best to recognize those who have helped provide me with valuable knowledge and assistance in bringing this book to its completion.

I want to especially thank Lois Brown for her expertise in research and editing. In addition, I want to thank the following health professionals for sharing their knowledge of noni with me. They include Dr. Bert Acosta, Alan Bailey, Bryant Bloss, M.D., Dr. Cliff Blumberg, Dr. Carlton Braitwaite, Robert Detrano, M.D., Richard T. Dicks, William Doell, D.O., Dr. Eiichi Furusawa, Dr. Brent Frame, Dr. Charles Garneir, Scott Gerson, M.D., Dr. Ernesto Gomez, Steven Hall, M.D., Dr. Jesse Hanley, the late Mona Harrison, M.D., Dr. Ralph Heinicke, Dr. Tomo Hiramatsu, Dr. Anne Hirazumi Kim, Dr. Patrick Joseph , Dr. Kay, Dr. Samuel Kolodney, Haruhiko Kugo, M.D., Peter Lodewich, M.D., Dr. Jim Marcoux, Dr. W.T. Meier, John Mike, M.D., Susan Mike, M.D., Dr. Joel Murphy, Richard Passwater, Ph.D., Orlando Pile, M.D., Dr. Nathan Rabb, Dr. Nelson T. Rivers, Larry Scott, Keith Sehnert, M.D., Allen Scheuneman, M.D., Dr. Rick T. Smith, Gary Tran, D.V.M., Dr. Thomas Velleff, and Mian-Ying Wang, M.D.

This book would never have seen the light of day if it hadn't been for the following visionaries who introduced TAHITIAN NONI® Juice to the world: Kerry Asay, Kim Asay, Kelly Olsen. Stephen Story, and John Wadsworth.

Next, I wish to thank Dru and Maeva White, Ken and Mary Roland, Gary and Ann Wilson, Mark and Jo Rose, Floyd and Ann Holdman, and Del and Sylvia Williams, for their perspective and genealogical help.

I also want to thank the following for their council and guidance: Kevin and Jenny Baadsgaard, John and Laurie Bentley, Andre and Françoise Blanchard, Dale Brenner, Lil Johnson, Usa Johnson, Susie and Caleb Kwok, Harold and Jesan Ledda, Dale Mahoney, Dave and Dianne Maxwell, Birger Oolvsson, Pat Patterson, Sal and Joan Serio.

Additionally, there are those who provided me with and/or helped me obtain many of the outstanding testimonials, some used in the book; these include: Doug Alcorn, Lynn Kathleen Ashcraft, J. Michelle Boykin, Bob and Della Bourke, Carlton and Joycie Braithwaite, Dave and Paulla Castle, Tsai Angela and Lori Chang, E.J. Maki and Siu-Linn Chong, Yalan Lin Chuang, Richard Cooper, Trudy Crow, Robert Dean, Buddy Delaney, Jim Dickson, John Dover, Robert Fechner, Gale, Deborah Gear, Glad Grand International People, Steve and Debra Gray, Marcus and Faith Howship, David Johnson, Gwen Kaese, Marie Mehner and Jack Kelly, Jeanette Komsi, Pat and Sawan Kongpat, Kathleen Gambino Labb, Ivy Way Lee, Sherri and Zachary Lipps, Frances Lowe, Joan L. Mailing, Tom and Elise Markham, Tom Matthews, Paul Miller, Ann Moran, Fay Nicholls-Holt, Ann Olavsson, David and Rosa Olivares, Chuck and Carol Parker, Paul and Margaret Pierce, Dan Ritchie, Joanne Ritter, Helen Rivers, Shannon and Dawn Roland, Karen Rzewnicki, Sal and Joan Serio, Michael Sossin, Terry Sowards, Tom and Manie Thornton, Michelle Titus, Katrina Tran, Jose Miguel Undurraga, Edgardo and Irma Valdivieso, Rob and Janine Witty, Bert and Helga Wolters, Wen Chi Wu, and Joleen Ziegler.

I could not have obtained international testimonials had it not been for the guidance which I received from Brett Barrett, Hector Contreras, John Calvert, Doug Castro, Sun Fu Chong, Cody Day, Lennart Engstrom, Scott Florence, David Garcia, Darrell Ieremia, Eduardo Krebsky, Carsten Marx, Seth Miller, Joseph Morton, Thorsten Mueller, Craig Richards, Thierry Sorhaitz, Phil Sykes,

Edouad Tuairau, Bryant Wadsworth, David Wadsworth, Kenny Wan, Phil Welch, Shon Whitney, and Peter Willden.

I owe many thanks to Jarakae Jensen for sharing his expert scientific and research knowledge about noni; to Pamela Beckham, for her gracious willingness to provide whatever assistance was asked of her; to Tom Black, Ben Tyler, Joel Neilsen, Aaron Garrity, Heather Maddison, Andre Peterson, Suzanne Tyler, Blaine Hawkes, and Harry Finkelstein, Brett West, and Kathy Wilson for their input and assistance in numerous matters; to Noni Blues singers Tommy Lyons, Mel Steeple, and Gary Romer for their inspirational songs about noni; to Parveez Shahviri for electronic advice; to Colby Allen and McKinley Oswald for their continued confidence and input into the project; to Frema Solomon, M.M.H., my agent and editor who also helped in so many ways.

I express my gratitude to Ken Dumas, Nancie J. Fleming, Miriam Glazer R.N., Cressa Goodman, Mike, Janice and Benjamin Goodman, Steve and Denise Goodman, Evalee Harrison, Evelyn Kryt, Chuck Layton, Priscilla Martinez, Tom and Adrian Mathews, Mindi Preston, Neil Reinhardt, Tom Corbett and Alina Rosiak, Priscilla Salazar, Gloria Schanely, Jack and Stella Shelburn, Amy Soratham, A. Warren and Laurelle Turski, John R. Wadsworth, Merlin and Bonnie Weekes and Camry for helping me better appreciate the value of noni.

Of course, this book would be incomplete without the feedback from over 1,227 Health Professionals representing over 25,314 individuals who were willing to share their accounts of how noni juice brought about a positive effect in their health and well-being. Again, I give many thanks to all those who contributed.

Amazing Noni Juice

During my over 30 years as a practicing medical professional, prescribing medication was relatively easy. Once the proper diagnosis was made, prescribing simply meant taking into consideration the different characteristics of the patient (i.e. severity of illness, gender, weight, age, allergies, etc.) and putting it in my mind's computer. Presto… the amount of medication was clear.

Since my retirement from the clinical practice of medicine, I have become more involved with natural healing. This has brought to my attention the ambiguity and confusion that exists when it comes to how much of a certain nutritional substance could or should be used in order to augment one's health. Suggested use of many nutritional supplements is many times based on trial and error, which over time and use, somewhat regulates itself.

I decided to find a plant with a proven track record of successes and with unique health benefits worthy of study. I was interested in finding out how much of it people took to help different conditions. This led me to the fruit of the Morinda citrifolia plant (noni). I soon found the people of the islands of the south pacific had used noni to promote healthy living for over 2,000 years. Noni flourishes in the lush and unspoiled islands of French Polynesia, of which the best known is Tahiti. On this tropical island, noni fruit is used to make TAHITIAN NONI® Juice. I spoke to the natives who harvest noni and who have long benefited from its use. I believe that for optimal effectiveness, noni juice should have the following characteristics: grown in a pollution-free, unspoiled tropical environment; harvested by natives who, from tradition, know when and how to pick it; and to be freshly processed and packaged under careful supervision in a way so as not to destroy its natural beneficial ingredients, or be contaminated. The noni product should contain no less than 90 percent pure, unadulterated noni juice, with each ounce containing between 9 to 17 calories, 2 to 4 grams of total carbohydrates, and no added additives. The noni should also be tested to be contaminant-free. Please see Table 1 for a complete listing of the major known nutraceuticals identified in noni.

Table 1. Nutraceuticals identified in noni

1-butanol
1-hexenol
1-methoxy-2-formyl-3-hydroxy
anthraquinone
2,5-undecadien-1-ol
2-heptan one
2-methyl-2-butanoyl decanoate
2-methyl-2-butanoyl hexanoate
2-methyl-3,5,6-trihydroxyanthraquinone-6-
§-primeveroside
2-methyl-3,5,6-trihydroxyanthraquinones
2-methyl butanoic acid
2-methylpropanoic acid
24-methylcycloartanol
24-methylene cholesterol
24-methylenecycloartanyl linoleate
3-hydroxyl-2-Butazone
3-hydroxymorindone
3-hydroxymorindone-6-§-primeveroside
3-methyl-2-buten-1-ol
3-methyl-3-buten-1-ol
3-methylthiopropanoic acid
5,6-dihydroxylucidin
5,6-dihydroxylucidin-3- §-primeveroside
5,7-acacetin7-O-§-D-(+)-gluco pyranoside
5,7-dimethylapigenin-4Õ-O-§-D-
D(+)=galactopyranoside
6,8-di methoxy-3-methyl anthraquinone-1, -
O-§-rhamnosyl
gluco pyranoside
6-dodecanoic-y-lactone
7-hydroxy-8-methoxy-2-methyl
anthraquinone
8,11,14-eicosatrienoic acid
acetic acid
alizarin
alkaloids
anthragallol 1,2-dimethyl ether
anthraquinones
anthragallol 2,3-dimethyl ether
asperuloside
benzoic acid
benzyl alcohol
butanoic acid
calcium

campesteryl glycoside
campesteryl linoleic glycoside
campesteryl palmitate
campesteryl palmityl glycoside
campesterol
carbonate
carotene
cycloartenol
cycloartenol linoleate
cycloartenol palmitate
damnacanthal
decanoic acid
elaidic acid
ethyl decanoate
ethyl hexanoate
ethyl octanoate
ethyl palmitate
eugenol
ferric iron
gampesteryl linoleate
glucose
glycosides
heptanoic acid
hexadecane
hexa-amide
hexanedioic acid
hexanoic acid
hexose
hexyl hexanoate
iron
isobutyric acid
iso caproic acid
iso fucosterol
isofucosteryl linoleate
isovaleric acid
lauric acid
limonene
linoleic acid
lucidum
lucidum-3- §-primeveroside
magnesium
methyl 3-methylthio-propanoate
methyl decanoate
methyl elaidate
methyl hexanoate

methyl octanoate
methyl oleate
methyl palmitate
morenone-1
morenone-2
morindadiol
morindanigrine
morindin
morindone
morindone-6-§-primeveroside
mucilaginous matter
myristic acid
n-butyric acid
n-valeric acid
nonanoic acid
nordamnacanthal
octadecanoic acid
octanoic acid
oleic acid
palmitic acid
paraffin
pectins
pentose
phenolic body
phosphate
physcion
physcion-8-O [[L-arabinopyranosyl] (1-3) {§-D- g-D- galactopyranosyl (1-6) {§-D- galactopyranoside}]]
potassium
protein

proxeronine
proxeroninease
resins
rhamnose
ricinoleic acid
rubiadin
rubiadin-1-methyl ether
scopoletin
sitosterol
sitosteryl glycoside
sitosteryl linoleate
sitosteryl linoleyl glycoside
sitosteryl palmitate
sitosteryl palmityl glycoside
sodium
sorandjidiol
§-sitosterol
stearic acid
sterols
stigmasterol
stigmasteryl glycoside
stigmasteryl linoleate
stigmasteryl linoleyl glycoside
stigmasteryl palmitate
stigmasteryl palmityl glycoside
terpenoids
trioxymethylanthraquinone
undecenoic acid
ursolic acid
xeronine

Taken with permission from Dr. Anne Hirazumi Kim's work and modified by author.

In the next chart, Table 2, you will find listed pertinent nutritional information specifically about TAHITIAN NONI® Juice.

Table 2. TAHITIAN NONI® Juice Nutritional Information

Ingredients: About 90 percent-reconstituted Morinda citrifolia fruit juice from pure juice puree from French Polynesia. About 10 percent pure natural grape and blueberry juice concentrate, balance blended with pure, natural flavors.

Vitamin and Mineral Content for One Serving (1 fluid ounce):

NUTRIENT	AMOUNT	% RDA‡
Vitamin A	5.88 IU	0.117%
Vitamin C	6.029 mg	10%
Calcium	6.76 mg	0.67%
Iron	0.1088 mg	0.6%
Vitamin E	0.235 IU	0.78%
Vitamin B1	0.0029 mg	0.196%
Vitamin B2	0.0029 mg	0.17%
Niacin	0.147 mg	0.735%
Vitamin B6	0.038 mg	1.91%
Folic Acid	7.35 mcg	1.84%
Vitamin B12	0.097 mcg	1.62%
Biotin	1.47 mcg	0.49%
Pantothenic Acid	0.147 mcg	1.47%
Phosphorus	2.058 mg	0.205%
Magnesium	3.088 mg	0.772%
Zinc	0.047 mg	0.313%
Copper	0.006 mg	0.294%

OTHER MINERALS	AMOUNT
Chromium	0.147 mg
Manganese	0.25 mg
Molybdenum	0.294 mg
Sodium	12.35 mg
Potassium	28.52 mg

Carbohydrate Content for One Serving (1 fluid ounce):

CARBOHYDRATE	AMOUNT
Fructose	1.2 grams
Glucose	1.1 grams
Fiber	0.7 grams

†There is essentially no fat or protein in noni juice.
‡Less than 2% of the RDA is not a significant source for this vitamin or mineral, so you don't have to worry about overdose.
Used with permission from Tahitian Noni International.

Noni is Safe

So much has been said in the media and medical community about the safety, or non-safety, of herbs and natural food supplements. When it comes to noni, specifically TAHITIAN NONI® Juice, put your mind at rest. TAHITIAN NONI® Juice has been tested to see if it contains more than 300 different toxins. Every test has come up negative. The juice itself goes through a thermal pasteurization that keeps it safe while allowing the special compounds within the juice to remain active.

In December of 2002, TAHITIAN NONI® Juice passed inspection by Europe's Novel Food Act Committee (much like the U.S. government's FDA in the United States). After rigorous testing, the European Committee approved the juice for sale as a novel food in Europe. It concluded, "There were no indications of adverse effects from laboratory animal studies on subacute and subchronic toxicity, genotoxicity, and allergenicity" from noni juice.

Other studies have observed animals and humans consuming up to seven bottles of noni juice a day with no adverse reaction. Of course, there may be some people or animals (and statistically speaking the chance is quite low) who are allergic to some of the ingredients in noni.

As for allergic reactions in animals, I refer to the expertise of Dr. Gary Tran. Dr. Tran is a veterinarian who has used noni with thousands of four-legged patients. In the thousands of animals that Dr. Tran has treated with noni, very few have had any negative reaction. He says he has only seen a few dogs have a severe itching reaction to TAHITIAN NONI® Juice. He believes the reaction is actually due to the grape or blueberries in the juice since an animal most likely has been exposed to these fruits before and not to noni. In the case of a severe allergic reaction, call the vet promptly and discontinue the use of this product. If there are minor allergic reactions present, stop the juice for three days and then begin again this time at half the dosage as before. Then slowly build up.[1]

No food product can ever honestly claim that is non-allergenic to 100 percent of the population. That is simply impossible. In some cases, minor allergic symptoms to noni may occur. This would include things such as belching, gas, mild transient diarrhea, or a slight rash or itching. If this is the case, reduce the amount of noni consumed until the undesired symptoms disappear. If these symptoms persist, stop drinking noni juice. In the case of a major allergic reaction (persistent diarrhea, hives, swelling, or difficulty in swallowing or breathing) stop drinking noni immediately. When all the symptoms disappear you may try drinking noni again at half the amount. If possible, slowly build back up to the more helpful amount. If any symptoms reappear, stop drinking noni juice. In both cases, notify your health professional and follow his or her advice.

Many also ask what sort of ph effect noni has on the body. To determine the pH of a metabolized food, it must be turned into ash by heating it to over 500 degrees. The extreme heat burns off the organic matter, and the leftover powder is made of mineral matter called ash. The ash is moistened with water and then the pH is measured. This remaining inorganic (or mineral) matter will determine whether that food raises (alkaline) or lowers (acidic) the pH of the blood once the food is metabolized by your body. In the case of noni, the pH of noni juice outside the body is 3.3 to 3.6 (acidic). However, when noni is metabolized in the body it has an alkaline effect on the blood.

Also, it's important to remember that the body has a buffering mechanism that is an inherent part of our physiology. When this buffering mechanism is working correctly, the amount of juice a person drinks may not make much difference on the ultimate pH of his or her blood.

The Noni Phenomenon

Before delving into each of the specific health conditions for which people benefit from using noni, I want to quickly summarize how I believe noni is able to help so many people with so many different health problems. While the working theory I am about to present does not cover the only reason noni is such an effective natural health supplement, I believe it does help explain why this ancient fruit is able to improve the symptoms of so many varied types of health problems.

One of the theories used to explain noni's health effects revolves around one of its putative main components—proxeronine. It is believed that once in the body, proxeronine travels to specific parts of cells, such as the mitochondria, microsomes, Golgi apparatus, reticuloendothelium, electron transport system, DNA, RNA, and etc. Within the cell, these components communicate with each other (intracellular), and with other cells (intercellular). It was established by Dr. Anne Hirazumi Kim that noni augments the release of high amounts of nitric oxide from immune cells.[2] I coupled her work with the work from the 1998 Nobel Prize winners in medicine who are Drs. Robert Fuchgott, Ferried Murad, and Louis Igano. These scientists demonstrated that nitric oxide in low concentrations allows cells to communicate with each other. Nitric oxide becomes one of their special languages.[3] The 1999 Nobel Prize was awarded to Rockerfeller University Biologist Dr. Guenther Blobel who explained how proteins are shipped to cells using a "postal and zip code" sort of system.[4] I believe when a person does not experience optimal health, it is because some cells are sick.[5]

Relying on research from other scientists, I have constructed my own theory about how the body is able to distribute the important biochemical compounds in noni. According to the theory, once in the body proxeronine travels to specific cells and settles in the cell's Golgi apparatus and reticuloendothelium. Within these structures, proxeronine combines with other natural biochemicals and building blocks (i.e. hormones, proteins, enzymes, serotonin, vitamins, minerals, and antioxidants) where it exerts its action. It is postulated the Golgi apparatus and the reticuloendothelium then assemble all the necessary compounds into a specific "package" and deliver the "package" to the parts of the cell, which are sick, or they may carry the "package" via the blood stream to other sick cells in other parts of the body. This is similar to how letters are sent to a specific address based upon the specified postal zip code.[6] The more science learns, the more we realize what a true phenomenon our bodies are. The way in which our bodies get the correct amounts of what we need to the right place at the right time is fascinating.

As the receiving sick cell opens the "package" sent by the Golgi apparatus and the reticuloendothelium, the packaged proxeronine combines with another cellular enzyme called proxeroninease. According to the research by Dr. Ralph Heinicke,[7] this combination converts into xeronine. Others believe that xeronine aids the cell to repair and regenerate itself. This is one way I believe that noni juice from Tahiti helps the body heal itself.

A simple illustration of this would be to compare proxeronine to that of a conductor of a symphony orchestra. Just as a conductor skillfully conducts the participants in an orchestra, proxeronine directs the various amounts of nutraceuticals, other natural biochemicals and building blocks (i.e. hormones, proteins, enzymes, serotonin, vitamins, minerals, antioxidants) to go to that part of the sick cell(s) to help in healthy regeneration. Once this happens, under the direction of its conductor, the cells once again work in harmony and play beautiful, helpful music.

One might logically ask why use noni juice from Tahiti to replenish proxeronine? Why not obtain it from food? The answer is simple. Noni is a food and is by far the richest known source of proxeronine. It has more than forty times more proxeronine than its closest competitor, pineapple. TAHITIAN NONI® Juice is among the purest that can be found in the world. It is grown and harvested in the pristine environment of French Polynesia and is routinely tested for over 600 contaminants by two independent laboratories. No contaminants have been found in TAHITIAN NONI® Juice.

Suggested Noni Usage

Ever since noni has become available in the United States, I have studied the tropical fruit, *Morinda citrifolia*. From my studies I have found some general guidelines on how much noni juice to drink to help some health situations. In other cases, many are still searching for guidance to figure out the optimal amount of TAHITIAN NONI® Juice to improve their specific health concerns.

In Table 3, I include general guidelines for a test, loading, optimal, and maintenance serving of noni juice. Animals under 100 pounds should drink the amount of noni recommended for children, and animals over 100 pounds should drink the amount suggested for adults. In addition, for every 50 pounds over 250 pounds, an extra one-half ounce of noni should be added to all recommended amounts for people and animals. I created these guidelines from results of an independent study done by researchers at the University of Illinois College of Medicine.[8]

Table 3. Average ounces of TAHITIAN NONI® Juice consumed by users

TEST SERVING: 3 DAYS

Adult (over 16 years)
      Before breakfast   1 tsp.
      Before dinner   1 tsp.

Child (under 16 years)
      Before breakfast   1 tsp.

LOADING SERVING: MONTH 1

Adult (over 16 years)
      Before breakfast   2 oz.
      Before dinner   2 oz.

Child (under 16 years)
      Before breakfast   1 oz.
      Before dinner   1 oz.

OPTIMAL SERVING: MONTH 2 THROUGH MONTH 6

Adult (over 16 years)
      Before breakfast   2 oz.
      Before dinner   1 oz.

Child (under 16 years)
      Before breakfast   1 oz.
      Before dinner   1/2 oz.

MAINTENANCE/PREVENTION SERVING: MONTH 7 AND AFTER

Adult (over 16 years)
      Before breakfast   1 oz.
      Before dinner   1 oz.

Child (under 16 years)
      Before breakfast   1 oz.

For simplicity, I call it the 4/3/2/ Plan: 4 ounces for the first month; 3 ounces for the next five months; and 2 ounces thereafter. Children, less than 16 years take half the amount.

In this book I have expanded on the above chart. I feel that if a person is suffering from one of the following 29 health conditions, the amount of noni juice he or she drinks should be calculated a little differently. My method for estimating a more "catered" type of suggested noni usage is based on the information that I gathered from more than 1,227 health professionals worldwide who have experience with TAHITIAN NONI® Juice. Their data represent more than 25,314 noni users as well as the health conditions from which they suffer. This information leads me to conclude that different ounces of noni juice help people with specific health conditions.

This information is summarized in Table 4 and Table 5. In Table 4 the "Total#" column represents the number of people who consumed noni juice for that specific condition, and the %Helped column gives the percentage of how many of those people reported they had positive results. Please see Tables 4 and 5 on the following pages.

Table 4. 29 Conditions Helped By People Who Drink Noni (n=25,314)

Information from over 1,227 health professionals representing over 25,314 noni juice drinkers from over 80 countries. An individual could mark more than one health condition for which he or she was drinking noni,

Condition, Decreased Symptoms	Total #	% Helped
1. Allergy	3,198	86 %
2. Arthritis	1,675	78 %
3. Asthma	8,077	71 %
4. Cancer	2,188	69 %
5. CFIDS, Fibromyalgia	3,524	77 %
6. Depression	1,512	80 %
7. Diabetics, Types 1 & 2	5,575	82 %
8. Digestion	3,171	90 %
9. Energy, increased	16,056	90 %
10. Heart Disease	2,158	76 %
11. High Blood Pressure, decreased	1,869	84 %
12. HIV	150	55 %
13. Immune System	3,707	77 %
14. Kidney Disease	3,764	67 %
15. Menstruation	3,798	79 %
16. Mental Acuity, increased alertness	5,543	73 %
17. Multiple Sclerosis	25	52 %
18. Muscle, increased body building	1,216	70 %
19. Obesity, lost some excess weight	5,526	72 %
20. Pain, including headaches	6,828	86 %
21. Parkinson's Disease	25	52 %
22. Respiratory Problems	3,857	72%
23. Skin and Hair Problems	877	78 %
24. Sexual Enhancement increased	2,984	84 %
25. Sleep, improved	2,025	75 %
26. Smoking, stopped	876	56 %
27. Stress, coped better	6,743	74 %
28. Stroke	1,806	53 %
29. Well-being, felt better	7,879	80 %

In Table 5, I report the minimum, average, and maximum amount of noni juice people drank who suffered from specific illnesses. I organized the 29 different health conditions into four groups that had the same averages. Please note that I did not include in my statistical analysis a few very extreme reported amounts of consumed noni juice that fell way out of the normal range. Also note that the averages are rounded to the closet 1/2 ounce.

Table 5. Breakdown of Ounces of Noni Consumed Per Day by Condition

Group 1: Min. 1/2 oz/day • Average Consumption 2 oz/day • Max. 21oz/day

Energy, increased
Mental Acuity, increased alertness
Muscle, increased bodybuilding
Sexual Enhancement
Skin and Hair Problems, improved
Stress, coped better
Well-being, felt better

Group 2: Min. 1/2 oz/day • Average Consumption 2 1/2 oz/day • Max. 24 oz/day

Allergy, lessened symptoms
Asthma, improved
Digestion, improved
Kidney Health, improved
Menstruation, lessened symptoms
Obesity, lost some excess weight
Sleep, improved

Group 3: Min. 1/2 oz/day • Average Consumption 3 oz/day • Max. 28 oz/day

Arthritis, lessened symptoms
Depression, lessened symptoms
Diabetes, Types 1&2, improved
High Blood Pressure, decreased
Pain, including headaches, decreased
Respiratory Problems, fewer symptoms
Smoking, stopped

Group 4: Min. 1/2 oz/day • Average Consumption 3 1/2 oz/day • Max. 30 oz/day
 Cancer, lessened symptoms
 CFIDS, Fibromyalgia, lessened symptoms
 Heart Disease, decreased symptoms
 HIV, lessened symptoms
 Immune System
 Multiple Sclerosis, lessened symptoms
 Stroke, decreased symptoms
 Parkinson's Disease
 Stroke, decreased symptoms

This "custom" usage chart may be helpful to those who are looking for a more precise amount of noni juice to drink according to the 29 different conditions that they wish to improve. Please remember that in some rare cases allergic symptoms to noni may occur. If persistent diarrhea or any major allergic symptoms appear, such as hives, swelling, or difficulty in swallowing or breathing, stop drinking noni for three days, then start drinking it again at half the amount. If possible, slowly build back up to the more helpful amount.

In each of the following 16 sections, I will cover the illnesses and conditions listed in Tables 4 and 5 in more detail. Specifically, I will cite the more common symptoms of the condition, its believed causes, how it noni juice may help those who suffer from the condition. I will address and how much noni juice others who have suffered from the condition have used to promote their health. In essence, I hope that you use the rest of this book as a quick reference for those who are seeking a more clearly researched path to enhance their health using a natural substance such as TAHITIAN NONI® Juice. In summary, the suggested testing and loading amounts of noni is found in Table 3. The amount of noni consumed each day by those people in my study who had successful outcomes for 29 different conditions is found and explained in Table 5.

The best amount of noni juice to drink is the amount that helps you the most!

Section One: Cancer

Simply put, cancer is a cellular malfunction. When suffering from cancer, the human body loses normal cellular controls, which results in the malignant cell's unregulated growth. These cancer cells have a lack of differentiation and invade local tissue, travel elsewhere, and metastasize. The disease itself begins by one cell that mutates or changes. The abnormal cell maintains that mutation through the cell's reproduction process despite the efforts of the human body's defense system, which tries to eliminate abnormal cells. These mutated cells (resulting from abnormal DNA) then travel through the body, setting up residency in one or more of the body's organs. There are now well over one hundred types of cancer that can exist within the human body.

Since there are so many types of cancer, each with their own abnormal DNA and different set of signs and symptoms, it is impossible in this short review to cover all of them. From my experience at the Johns Hopkins Hospital, the single most common symptom that I observed was the loss of energy. I also observed in many different types of cancer such abnormalities as skin discoloration, and non-healing sores, detectable lumps under the skin, elevated temperature and weight loss. These are often associated with many other signs and symptoms. Most types of cancer start subtly and can only be properly diagnosed early on by having regular medical check ups and specific testing. The earlier a cancer is detected and treated, the better the outcome.

I believe noni's effect on cancer most likely deals with the fact that both noni and cancer work on a cellular level. It is further believed that noni enhances cellular structure while cancer, of course, destroys it. One of noni's key components, proxeronine, is sent to "sick" cells within the body by the Golgi apparatus and reticuloendothelium. I believe that these sick cells attract proxeronine and an enzyme, proxeroninease. The interaction creates xeronine, a cellular enhancer. A longer description of this is given in the section "Amazing Noni Juice."

Several other studies have been performed in laboratories in order to validate *Morinda citrifolia's* cancer-fighting abilities. In one such study, four Japanese scientists injected ras cells (cells that are precursors to many malignant growths) with a substance called damnacanthal found in *Morinda citrifolia*. They observed that the injection of damnacanthal significantly inhibited the ras cells from reproducing.[9] Proxeronine and damnacanthal are substances within *Morinda citrifolia* that are believed to be anti-cancer agents. In addition, research has revealed that noni helps stimulate the body's production of other cancer-fighting elements such as nitric oxide, interleukins, interferon, tumor necrosis factor, lipopolysaccharides, and natural killer cells.

It is believed by some that *Morinda citrifolia* might exert a preventive and protective action against cancer during the initiation stage, which is the first phase of the formation of cancer. A study performed by Mian-Ying Wang, M.D., at the University of Illinois College of Medicine at Rockford, showed that mice who were given a solution of 10 percent noni juice for a week and then injected with DMBA, a known cancer-causing agent, had significantly lower DNA adduct markers (a test for abnormal DNA) than DMBA-injected mice fed only water. The lower the number of DNA adduct markers, the more protection against cancer. The noni-fed mice had 50 percent fewer DNA markers in the lungs than the water-fed mice without TAHITIAN NONI® Juice, 60 percent fewer markers in the heart, 70 percent fewer in the liver, and 90 percent fewer in the kidneys. Therefore, TAHITIAN NONI® Juice gave the greatest protection from cancer to the kidneys (90 percent) and the least protection to the lungs (50 percent). Please see Figures 1 and 2.[10]

Figure 1. Density of DNA adduct markers in kidney and heart

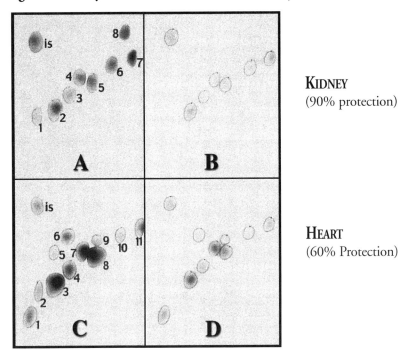

KIDNEY
(90% protection)

HEART
(60% Protection)

Autoradiographic density pattern of DNA adduct markers (single nucleotide) from two-dimensional thin layer chromatography. *These figures show that the density of the markers of the group of rats who took noni as seen on the right side (Band D) is significantly lower than the density of the markers of the group on the left (A and C) who did not drink noni. The lower the density , the more the prevention and protection against cancer.*

Figure 2. Density of DNA adduct markers in liver and lung

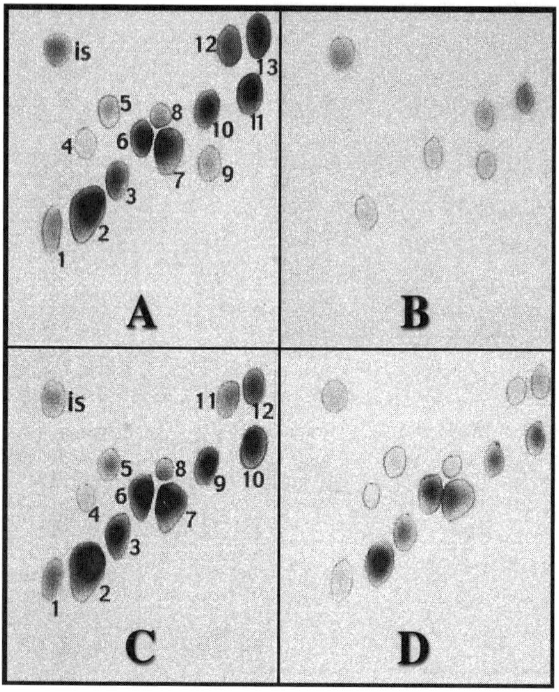

LIVER
(70% protection)

LUNG
(50% protection)

A summation of the latest study done by Dr. Wang and her associate can be seen in Table 6. Dr. Wang's study addresses the hypothesis of whether or not TAHITIAN NONI® Juice possesses a cancer preventative effect at the initiation stage of carcinogenesis. Preliminary data indicates that pre-treatment for one week with TAHITIAN NONI® Juice in drinking water at a concentration of 10% was able to prevent DMBA-DNA adduct formation (marker for developing cancer) in rats.[11]

Table 6. Pretreatment with rats drinking 10% noni juice from Tahiti

% CANCER REDUCTION (MALES)		% CANCER REDUCTION (FEMALES)
Heart	60%	30%
Lungs	50%	41%
Liver	70%	42%
Kidney	90%	80%

[Figures 1 and 2 and Table 6 were obtained from Dr. Mian-Ying Wang's work and are used here with her permission. Under no circumstances can these figures (or any portions of this book) be photocopied or duplicated in any way without written permission from the publisher.]

TAHITIAN NONI® Juice has proven antioxidant ability. This means it binds with or ties up the free radicals present within the body. Free radicals can damage cells that may lead to the cell's mutation to a cancerous cell. Many feel the antioxidant activity is an important function of noni juice and one of the reason so many people have reported success with fighting cancer using the juice. Table 7 shows how TAHITIAN NONI® Juice measures up in antioxidants compared with other well-known substances. In these results, TAHITIAN NONI® Juice is considered the "standard" or the substance to which all the other substances were measured against.

Table 7. Antioxidant Activity (LPO and TNB)

LPO = Lipid hydroperoxide quenching activity assay
TNB = Tetrazolium nitroblue, scavenger activity assay

Noni juice from Tahiti	100% (the standard)
Vitamin C	2.8 X Less
Pycnogenol®	1.4 X Less
GSP	1.1 X Less

Out of the 25,314 noni users in my survey, 2,188 suffered from some type of cancer. From this number, 69 percent of them reported positive health benefits after taking TAHITIAN NONI® Juice.

Amount of Noni Usage: The average amount consumed by the 69 percent who reported positive results was 3.5 ounces each day.

Also in my research, I came across a "noni recipe" that has been used by cancer patients who want to give their bodies an extreme boost. The "recipe" comes from a medical professional colleague, Orlando Pile, M.D. It is as follows:

1 bottle of TAHITIAN NONI® Juice a day for four days
1/2 bottle of TAHITIAN NONI® Juice a day for the next four days
8 ounces of TAHITIAN NONI® Juice a day for the next 30 days
3.5 ounces or resume your usual amount

"I Feel Better Than I Have in Years!"—Frances Lowe

"My name is Frances Lowe. I am 50 years old. Noni juice is an answer to my prayers! It is working wonderfully for me as part of my protocol to overcome advanced aggressive adenocarcinoma of the endometrium, which is cancer of the lining of the womb. I had been extremely ill since August 1998, suffering severe lower pelvic pain daily for 8 months, anemia from excessive loss of blood, and enduring doctors' misdiagnoses until Thursday, February 25, 1999, when I was brought to UCSD medical hospital in San Diego as a medical emergency.

"The wonderful staff of doctors and nurses there saved my life. During my stay in the hospital, I received the shattering news: aggressive endometrial cancer. The pathology report March 5,

---

1999, said, `grade 3 adenocarcinoma of the endometrium... at least a stage IIIC tumor.'

"In January 1999, my friends Chuck and Carol Parker brought me noni juice. When I was able to drink 2 ounces of noni juice, I noticed I did not need as much pain medication. While in the hospital, my husband brought noni juice to me and gave it to me with the doctor's permission (after all, simple fruit juice is not going to hurt). Several of the nurses surprised me when they said they also took TAHITIAN NONI® Juice.

"When I came home from the hospital, I suffered from nausea caused by the pain pills I was given. Five days later, I stopped taking the pain medication and started taking larger amounts of noni juice. The nausea stopped after several days and I haven't needed any pain medication since then.

"In April 1999, the doctors said I needed radiation treatments to the entire pelvic area and to the middle above my waist (because the involved lymph node was from this area). I declined the radiation treatment at that time, convinced that I needed to strengthen my body to fight this cancer, praying that God would heal me or bring me a treatment that would not have such extreme side effects.

"On April 14, 1999, I started taking 1 ounce of noni every hour with 5 ounces of water for a total of 24 ounces of noni and more than a gallon of water a day, for four days. I reduced this to 12 ounces TAHITIAN NONI® Juice per day for four more days and then to 8-10 ounces noni per day through July. I continued drinking nearly a gallon of water every day. On August 3, 1999, lab reports indicated that my body had mounted the fight against the cancer. My doctor was surprised that my liver function was so good, and he said I'm doing very well.

> *"I feel better than I have in years doing things such as: swimming, walking, lifting my 34-pound grandson, and singing in church and at home. I have a great appetite now, overflowing joy and lots of energy. My weight is stable at 127 pounds since April. My hair, which had shed terribly after my surgery, has grown back thicker than before, thanks to noni! I know that taking large amounts of noni juice in April helped turn my health around. I now take 6-8 ounces of noni juice per day. Noni is an important part of my natural food and supplements treatment program. I hope others have such wonderful results as I am having. I thank God for restoring my health and for creating noni!"*

One thing that I learned from people who reported that their cancer symptoms were helped by drinking noni, was that the best amount for them was the amount which helped them the most. Many people with very difficult problems were helped when they figured out the total amount of noni juice that helped each day, and then they drank it in divided amounts, hourly. Some did best by drinking one-half ounce of noni juice each hour while awake. Others did well by drinking one ounce an hour. Some people preferred drinking two ounces or more per hour. Drinking hourly amounts of noni was reported to have given relief not only to many people with cancer symptoms, but people suffering from other conditions listed in this book reported that the hourly method helped as well.

Section Two: Arthritis

Under the general umbrella term of "arthritis" lie many different kinds of diseases that result in pain associated with bodily movement. In fact, there are more than 100 different types of rheumatic diseases that are often misdiagnosed as arthritis. A short list of such diseases includes bursitis, tendinitis, systemic lupus, and connective and soft tissue diseases. Regardless of which disease one may suffer from, chronic pain is often his or her constant companion.

Common arthritis, called either osteoarthritis (OA) or degenerative joint disease (DJD), is found in the joints of the body, the most common areas being the knees and fingers. These joints become inflamed and sore from continued wear and tear. The cartilage that normally cushions the joints degenerates, leaving the raw joints to rub against each other. Often a person's condition exacerbates with age because of continued wear and tear.

Rheumatoid arthritis, on the other hand, can attack at any age and can affect your whole body. That is why it is called a systemic disease. It is an autoimmune disease that causes the body to destroy bodily tissues as if they were foreign invaders. Symptoms of rheumatoid arthritis include mild to severe joint dysfunction, fever, weight loss, stiffness, aching and loss of energy. Many times there is a red, painful lump located around the rheumatoid joint. In one form of autoimmune disease associated with arthritis, Sjögren's syndrome, the eyes and mouth may become very dry because the salivary glands are also affected.

In recent years some exciting studies have been published that shed light on how to more safely combat arthritis. The disease boils down to the body's over production of an enzyme called the COX 2 enzyme.

There are actually two COX enzymes in the body. They are COX 1 and COX 2. COX 1 is called the good COX enzyme, while COX 2 has earned the unflattering name as the bad enzyme. COX 1 is easily identifiable and is important in regulation cell function. COX 2, on the other hand, is generally undetectable in most tissues, but increases to high levels during acute inflammation. The COX 1 enzyme, or good enzyme, creates prostaglandins that protect the stomach lining and other parts of the body. The COX 2 enzyme creates prostaglandins that cause inflammation in the joints, muscles and other areas. The good COX 1 gene was found and identified on Chromosome 2; the COX 2 gene on Chromosome 9.

COX 1 is essential for blood clotting and for protecting the stomach. COX 2 is the key player in inflammation, pain, and fever. Nonsteroidal anti-inflammatory drugs (NSAIDs) and other arthritis medication steeply decrease the body's production of both enzymes, thereby decreasing inflammation while at the same time causing harm through loss of protection to the stomach and its lining. The ideal situation would be to find a substance that inhibited COX 2 but which did not significantly affect COX 1. There is such a substance and it is TAHITIAN NONI® Juice.

Researchers at an independent research facility found that indeed TAHITIAN NONI® Juice was a selective inhibitor of COX 2. In addition, the juice did little, if any, damage to the COX 1 enzyme. When scientists compared the TAHITIAN NONI® Juice COX 2 inhibition ratio to the COX 2 inhibition ratio of prescription arthritis medications, they found that TAHITIAN NONI® Juice compared "very favorably" to the prescription medications. Yet, TAHITIAN NONI® Juice exhibited none of the negative side effects that the prescription medications are known to cause. Next, researchers compared the TAHITIAN NONI® Juice COX 2 inhibition ratio to the COX 2 inhibition ratio of NSAIDs. In this category, TAHITIAN NONI® Juice far out-performed the over-the-counter medications. And again, the noni did not exhibit any of the negative side effects associated with NSAIDs.[12]

There are several other ways in which noni may alleviate the undesirable symptoms of arthritis. Pain is the number one complaint with arthritis. A laboratory in France conducted a study that showed mice, given a liquid form of *Morinda citrifolia,* had significantly increased reaction time to a hot plate. The researchers concluded that this experiment demonstrated noni's analgesic qualities.[13] Next, *Morinda citrifolia* has also been shown to contain scopoletin, which has anti-inflammatory and histamine-inhibiting effects, both of which are excellent for the promotion of smooth joint movement. Finally, the cellular enhancing qualities of noni may also minimize the damage to the joints and other involved tissues.

An incredible 78 percent of the 1,675 people with either osteoarthritis or rheumatoid arthritis in my survey reported lessened symptoms after starting a regimen of TAHITIAN NONI® Juice.

<u>Amount of Noni Usage:</u> The average amount consumed by the 78 percent who reported positive results was 3 ounces per day.

"I'm Without Pain…"—Ed, a 44-year-old Sufferer of Ankylosing Spondylitis (A Form of Arthritis)

"I am a Registered Massage Therapist in Ontario Canada. I see over 40 patients a week. My greatest concern for my patients is their health. If you do not have your health, you have nothing. Since introducing my patients to noni, I have seen remarkable and significant results.

"I have been massaging a 44-year-old man once a month for a year and a half with a condition called Ankylosing Spondylitis. This is a condition where the spine and hipbone meet, and the spinal column calcify and fuse together along with the vertebral bodies. The same process can take place between the neck and head. This is classified as a form or arthritis. With this fusing, the

---

person is stiff and there is no flexibility in the spine. If you were to take an x-ray, you would see why the condition is also referred to as `Bamboo spine' and `Marie Strumpell's Disease.' This condition starts on both sides and moves slowly up the spine. It is very important that the patient keep the head looking straight ahead. If they do not and the head is looking down, the neck will fuse in the flexed position. There will be little or no turning the neck.

"When Ed first came to me his complexion was gray, his face was somewhat wrinkled, his shoulders were rounded and his neck was flexed a little as he looked on the floor. It was hard for him to straighten up to look at me in the eyes. One month after his last visit he came through the door smiling away like a Cheshire cat. I noticed his complexion was clear with rosy cheeks and the most significant thing that was so noticeable was his posture. He was straighter with his shoulders back and his head was a lot straighter too. I said, 'Ed, what have you been doing? You look great!' He just stood there grinning. I kept asking him what he had been doing. Finally, he said 'I'm without pain for the first time in my life since I've been a teenager!' He said he had started taking something called TAHITIAN NONI® Juice.

" 'Ed,' I said, 'this is great news! You're getting your health back.' Ed told me that he was up on the roof laying shingles that day. (This is unheard of for a person who has this condition because he or she has to physically bend to do this job.) Ed said he started by taking 4 ounces of TAHITIAN NONI® Juice day. Ed said when he wakes up every morning, he is constantly smiling and his wife wants to know why. Ed said he replies, 'I don't know, I just am. I'm out of pain.'

"During the massage, I noticed a significant change in his spine. It did not feel the same as other times. It was more defined and you could feel where the lamina groove was situated where you never could before. It has now been five weeks since I have seen Ed. Today he came back for another treatment. This time he was much straighter. He said he had gone to the doctor and the doctor noticed how much straighter he was and how easily he moved out of the chair. What a change!"

Section Three: Fibromyalgia and Energy

Until about fifteen years ago, many medical professionals did not recognize Fibromyalgia as an actual disease. In fact, up to that time it was not politically correct for Fibromyalgia awareness groups to spread the word about the syndrome in medical conferences. In the last several years, more and more studies have been published that substantiate Fibromyalgia and chronic fatigue and immune dysfunction syndrome (CFIDS) as much more than just psychological problems, (as they were once incorrectly classified.) Researchers at the University of Alabama have discovered that patients with Fibromyalgia have abnormalities in the brain and central nervous system. For example, Fibromyalgia patients have significantly less blood flow to the parts of the brain that deal with pain, and they have twice the level of the brain chemical called Substance P, which helps nervous system cells communicate with each other about painful stimuli.[14] In other words, you feel more pain with Fibromyalgia.

Women are more likely than men to have Fibromyalgia and CFIDS, though the reason for this is not yet known. In fact, one study cited that 90 percent of Fibromyalgia sufferers are women.

Some of the more common symptoms of the disease are "all-over" chronic pain, trouble sleeping, stiffness, severe fatigue, memory loss, and extreme headaches.

The way in which noni may help those suffering from these two debilitating diseases is not exactly clear, however there are several possibilities. For instance, an increase in energy after taking TAHITIAN NONI® Juice was reported by 90 percent of the 16,056 people in my survey who were drinking noni juice. Those reported results are astounding. Since many fibromyalgia and CFIDS folks suffer from a loss of energy, an increase in energy from noni is a very positive side effect from the juice. However, there seems to be more going on than just an increase of energy. Currently researchers are experimenting with medication to increase blood flow to the brain (cerebral blood flow). Noni allows the body to produce more nitric oxide, which has clinically been shown to improve blood flow.[15]

From my study, of the 3,524 noni users that suffered from Fibromyalgia and CFIDS, 77 percent of them reported lessened symptoms after taking noni juice.

Amount of Noni Usage: The average amount consumed by the 77 percent who reported a positive result was 3.5 ounces a day.

"I Am Ready to Live the Second Half of My Life"— **Kathleen Gambino Labb**

"1972—I began experiencing symptoms of fatigue, depression, pain, headaches, and migraines. I sought help many times and was told it was stress. The symptoms would abate to some degree then reappear with greater severity for periods of months.

"January 1983—I had just graduated from college at the age of 39 with four children, a part-time job and an abusive husband. I became very physically ill and had a major depressive episode. Again I sought help from several different doctors to no avail. I was basically told, 'it is all in your head.'

"July 1983—I was diagnosed with biological depression by Dr. Norman Moss in Newton, Massachusetts. I was put on medication (Elavil 200 mg.) and I improved dramatically.

"1985 to 1992—During this time I experienced sporadic and extreme symptoms of fibromyalgia, palpitations, and liver abnormalities. Despite my constant bad health, I finished a degree at Harvard Divinity School.

"June 1993—After graduating from Harvard, the migraines were so debilitating I was desperate for relief. I turned to alternative methods, went off all my medications and proceeded to go down hill and become severely depressed. I also had pain everywhere and was completely exhausted.

"November 1994—I was in such pain, I could hardly walk and was so exhausted I could hardly get up off the couch. I finally called Dr. George Cohen, a rheumatologist at Massachusetts General Hospital. He was the first doctor to ever listen to all of my symptoms. He diagnosed the fibromyalgia and prescribed Elavil to add to the antidepressants I was taking (Trazodone and Wellbutrin). My symptoms marginally reduced with medication, but flared up with any stress. Occasionally I would have a few days of respite from some of my symptoms. During those times I felt like myself again, clear thinking, energetic, little pain, and even some joy. With my newfound energy, I would try to catch up on everything, and in a few days I would be totally exhausted.

"January 2, 1996—I had a frightening episode of getting complete-ly lost going to my homeopath (an easy twenty-minute ride from my home). I finally had to call him and have him talk me back to his office. I had been traveling for almost an hour, but had no sense of time or place. This is not the first incident of severe confusion or the last. In February 1999 I again got completely lost going to my gyne-cologist. By the time that I got to her office, I was shaking and my blood pressure was 169/110 (normal is 120/80). I shook for the rest of the day. After the episode in January of 1996, I consulted numer-ous doctors including: Fibromyalgia Specialist Dr. Goldenberg at Newton/Wellesley; Physiologist Dr. Christopher Quinn at Newton/Wellesley PT; Fibromyalgia/Allergies Specialist Dr. Carol Englender at Newton, MA; and Neurologist Dr. James Lehrich at Mass General Hospital. These specialists helped my condition improve some, but I still felt I was living a marginal existence.

"June 1997—There was a family crisis that caused me a great deal of stress. Subsequently, I became ill again with the symptoms of fibromyalgia. By August of 1997, I was severely ill with a high fever, sore throat, and extreme exhaustion. In late October, I was finally given a blood test and diagnosed with mono and acute strep-tococcus infection, which caused a rash all over my body. By then my liver was enlarged, I was dehydrated and in very bad shape.

"By February of 1999, I was ripe to try some other resource when a friend sold me a bottle of TAHITIAN NONI® Juice. Three days after starting noni I slept through the night. My sleeping disorder began at age six; it is one of the symptoms of fibromyalgia. At first I thought that this must be a placebo effect. After the fifth night of wonderful sleep I decided that I didn't care what it was, I was never going to go without my daily dose of noni again. Just five days before I was complaining to my doctor about my sleepless nights and he told me that it was just part of my disorder.

[Author's note: Just as this writer indicates she would not stop taking noni juice, an amazing 69 percent of all noni juice users interviewed said they too would not stop taking their noni juice because of the health benefits they experienced.]

"Two weeks after I started taking TAHITIAN NONI® Juice I had less pain overall and my energy increased dramatically to a level I had not felt in years. My mood was vastly improved, my colon and bladder symptoms disappeared, and my mind became sharper and my voice stronger. I continued to improve with each day. I usually note these changes with an epiphany. `I can move my wrists!' Looking out the car window with a moonrise on one side and a sunset on the other, I suddenly realized, `I can turn my neck from side to side!' It was a triumph the day I came out of the shower announcing that I could wash my own hair without pain or fatigue! These were small but important milestone for me!

"This weekend I was able to ride eight hours each way to and from Philadelphia and sit through a whole conference. We arrived home at 12:30 a.m. and got up Sunday and drove to Boston (over an hour each way), to another five-hour meeting. This would have been unthinkable just one month ago. A two-hour trip would normally leave me exhausted and in tremendous pain, and it would have taken me days to recover. This morning I woke up feeling great with almost no pain and with plenty of energy. These changes and many more have given me confidence that had diminished with the debilitating effects of the fibromyalgia. I am ready to live the second half of my life as I never lived before."

Section Four: Diabetes

Many people are surprised to learn that this nation's third top killer is diabetes, falling behind only heart disease and cancer. Fortunately, many of the effects of diabetes can be controlled. While there is no cure for the disease, studies show that by keeping one's blood sugar as close to normal as possible significantly reduces diabetes' long-term complications such as heart attacks, kidney failure, and blindness.

A diabetic's body is not able to properly turn food into energy. The cause of the problem is the body's proper production and use of the hormone called insulin. Beta cells in the pancreas manufacture insulin. There are two types of diabetes: Type I and Type II. In Type I diabetes, the body produces little or no insulin. It is often referred to as juvenile diabetes because it usually starts at a younger age and is more severe. In Type II diabetes the body produces enough insulin, (sometimes even too much). However, the insulin is unable to adequately enter the body's cells to break down sugar into energy. In a Type II diabetic, the body also has trouble properly utilizing fats and protein. Type II is the more common type, accounting for nearly 90 percent of all diabetics. It used to be referred to as "maturity-onset" diabetes.

Type I and Type II diabetes share some similar symptoms. The most common of which include: lack of energy, increased hunger, weight loss for Type I and weight gain for Type II, frequent urination, excessive thirst, blurred vision, nausea, abdominal pain, irritability, and weakness. While we do know that diabetes is genetic, or is passed on from generation to generation, scientists are not exactly sure of the precise cause except that the disease may be the result of a malfunction in the body's endocrine and immune systems.

Research has shown that if the immune system starts to turn on itself—perhaps the result of an autoimmune disorder—it may cause a complete obliteration of the pancreas' beta cells or at least a reduction in the number of functioning beta cells. This then affects the amount, purity, and effectiveness of the body's insulin. However, if the immune system is able to ward off an attack, the integrity of the body's insulin will be maintained.

More refined tests now make it possible to detect faulty immune antibodies in the blood well in advance of a person showing symptoms of diabetes. In some adults, these destructive antibodies may be present years before diabetic symptoms appear. This lag time is known as the "prediabetic stage." This prediabetic state, or destructive antibody producing state, can be found in other endocrine diseases such as Hashimoto's Thyroiditis, and Addison's Disease (adrenal insufficiency). Co-existing Thyroiditis and Addison's disease is called Schmidt's Syndrome.

In the 1960s, I was on the faculty of Medicine at the Johns Hopkins Medical School and a member of a medical team that researched Schmidt's Syndrome. The team was made up of many fine Johns Hopkins Hospital physicians such as the late Dr. A.M. Harvey, who was Chairman and Professor of the Department of Medicine; Dr. Ivan L. Bennett, who was Professor and Chairman of the Department of Pathology; Dr. Charles C. Carpenter, Chief Resident on the Osler Medical Service of the Johns Hopkins Hospital; and others. Our team found that many patients with Schmidt's Syndrome not only had antibodies targeted against the adrenal and thyroid glands but also against the insulin producing beta cells of the pancreas. We published the interrelationship between antibodies and the adrenal, thyroid and pancreas in peer-reviewed medical journals.[16,17]

I believe that one of noni's effects is on the pancreas and immune system. Current studies have revealed that noni may help modulate a healthy immune system by either enhancing an already functioning system or by stimulating the components of a sluggish one. In addition, as described earlier, noni is believed to fortify and maintain cell structure. This can be accomplished by noni acting as an adaptogen that can aid "sick" cells in repairing themselves. This could apply to diabetes by either helping malfunctioning beta cells in the pancreas or by aiding the cells that are unsuccessfully trying to receive and use the glucose from the blood.

Finally, drinking noni may also help relieve diabetic symptoms through its ability to stimulate the body's production of scopoletin and the indirect production of nitric oxide. Both may also be important factors in decreasing symptoms such as poor circulation and vision problems.

Since the intake of sugars—even natural sugars—may be important to track in a diabetic's diet, it is good to note that 4 ounces of noni juice equals one fruit exchange. A general rule for diabetics is to gradually start using noni juice. Keep in mind, however, since noni is a natural food it is no more likely to change a person's blood sugar level than any other fruit juice. Keeping a daily log of your blood sugar level is the best way to monitor any changes that perhaps may occur. A good recommendation is to check your blood sugar first thing in the morning (a fasting level) and then check it again in the late afternoon (around 4 p.m.). This will show how your body is metabolizing sugar and responding to the noni juice or anything else you have consumed.

Please note that a Type 1 diabetic should never substitute noni juice for insulin shots. A Type I diabetic may be able to reduce his or her insulin. Using a natural supplement such as noni juice should be done under the supervision of a doctor.

In my survey, of the 5,575 people who consumed noni juice for help with their diabetic symptoms, 82 percent of them reported that their diabetic symptoms lessened.

Amount of Noni Usage: The average amount consumed by the 82 percent who reported positive results was 3 ounces a day.

"One Happy Person"—Karen Rzewnicki

"I've been an insulin-dependent diabetic (Type 1) for more than 29 years. I currently take three injections daily and have done so for over 10 years. I test my blood sugars four times a day. I'm far from what you would call "controlled." Traditionally, my blood sugar has been very high (200 to 300+) with an occasional extreme low. I've tested as low as 23 while coming out of unconsciousness or a diabetic coma. "Normal" blood sugars for me would be 150 to 180, when I could get those numbers, though most doctors and laboratories wouldn't call that normal. Normal fasting sugar for most people is 70 – 110 mg/Dl. Needless to say, my diabetes hasn't been a fun ride.

"I am now in week five of taking noni according to Gene Dillman's recommendations. I am in week two of taking 4 ounces a day. I have had only one occasion of extremely low blood sugar during this time. My overall readings are more significant: they are much more balanced than they've ever been! I still have an occasional high, but most of my readings are much more acceptable than before. Numbers from 120 to 180 are much more frequent than before. And this has to be due to the noni because nothing else has changed—my activity level, my diet, nothing. If things continue this well, I'll be one happy person at the end of that time period."

Section Five: Asthma, Respiratory Problems, and Allergies

For those who suffer from severe asthma, easy tasks such as walking up the stairs or participating in an outdoor picnic can result in hours of labored breathing. Asthma is a chronic condition that affects more than 17 million Americans, and it is a condition that is growing. Studies show that the number of asthma cases in America has increased by 75 percent between the years 1980 and 1994. In addition, 90 percent of the deaths from asthma occur in the elderly, the majority of whom are women.[18] Most asthma deaths are preventable.

In an asthmatic person's lungs, the airways called bronchioles constrict abnormally when stimulated by things such as allergens, infections, and exercise, which makes it difficult to expel air from the lungs. Research has linked the presence of allergies with asthma, though not all asthmatics have allergies, and not all allergic people have asthma. Some of the main symptoms of the condition are wheezing, breathlessness, inability to exhale properly, a phlegm or mucus-producing cough, and loss of energy. Inflammation of the lungs is present even in mildest cases of asthma and can lead to other problems such as respiratory infections.

Genetic susceptibility seems to be one of the major culprits behind asthma. However, there are identifiable triggers of the condition. Asthma may be brought on by an allergic response, exercise, bacterial and viral infections, hormones, stress, and other triggers. One interesting note is that 30 to 40 percent of women experience a fluctuation in their asthma symptoms during their menstrual cycles.

Whatever it is that triggers a person's asthma, a food supplement such as noni juice may help in reducing the severity of the symptoms by boosting and modulating the immune system and enhancing the cellular structure of the bronchioles. This is, I believe, mostly due to the proxeronine bundled packages sent by the Golgi apparatus and reticuloendothelium to the affected "sick" cells.

My survey showed that in addition to asthma, general allergy symptoms (such as running nose, itchy eyes, hives, and even eczema) were reduced in those people who drank noni. Other, non-asthmatic respiratory illnesses have also responded to noni. Infections of the lungs, bronchitis, and pneumonia are all illnesses that affect people who do not have asthma. Pneumonia, for example, can be caused by thirty different causes. The five most common are bacteria, viruses, mycoplasmas, infectious agents such as fungi, and various chemicals. Since noni works on a cellular level, regardless of the causes of pneumonia, noni has the ability to strengthen weakened lung cells and boost the body's ability to naturally ward off the causative agents.

In my survey, of the 8,077 people who consumed noni juice for help with their asthmatic symptoms, 71 percent reported their symptoms lessened. In addition, of the 3,857 people who took noni for other non-asthma related respiratory problems, 72 percent reported improved health. An incredible 86 percent of the 3,198 noni drinkers with common allergies also reported a decrease in symptoms.

Amount of Noni Usage: The average amount consumed by the 71 percent who reported positive results with asthma symptoms was 2.5 ounces per day. The average amount consumed by those with other respiratory problems was 3 ounces per day. The average amount consumed by those with positive results with allergies was 2.5 ounces per day.

"He Does Not Need Inhalers Anymore"—Katrina Tran

"My son had asthma since he was two years old. Besides everyday medication, he also used two different types of inhalers. He coughed all the time, he was always short of breath, and he would start having an asthma attack every time he overplayed with other kids. He had to go to visit his specialist doctor very often for the asthma treatments. There were a few times that my husband and I thought we had to take him to the emergency room because it got so severe.

"As a mother, it's very difficult to see your child in pain and there's nothing you can do to help ease the pain. I felt so useless. The condition lasted longer than a year until May of this year, when a friend, Joleen Ziegler, introduced me to noni juice. After doing some research on this product, I let my son use it. He started with 1 ounce every morning and night. After two weeks I saw a lot of improvements in him. He did not have asthma attacks; he coughed less and spent more time playing with his friends and cousins. The second month I took him back to see his doctor for a check up. The doctor told me he was perfectly fine. For three months now, after using the noni juice, he does not need any more inhalers or cough medicine.

"Noni is part of our lives now. We all take one to 2 ounces a day just to maintain good health. This is truly a gift from God. Where else can you find something that works so well? Try it, experience it and you will see."

Section Six: Depression

"Noni Juice Helped Me Get Back Control over My Life"—
David Johnson

"My name is David Johnson; I am 38-years-old. I am an insulin dependent diabetic since the age of four. I was diagnosed as an asthmatic 15 years ago. Two years ago I developed angina, which is insufficient blood flow from the heart to meet the needed demand for oxygen. Six months later I had an angioplasty to help my heart disease. A balloon was inserted that opened the clogged arteries going to my heart. Three months after that I had a four-bypass open-heart surgery. This surgical procedure bypasses the blocked coronary artery and re-establishes blood flow to the heart.

"While my main artery blockages have been by-passed, many of my small arteries supplying blood to my heart are also blocked. The medical profession can do nothing to reverse this condition. I have never let my health issues get me down, and I have lived an extremely full life. However, being a young married man with four young children, having doctors tell me that there is no hope, has led me to times of depression. It left me wondering if it is worth continuing the struggle to live, as my quality of life was slipping through my fingers.

"About two months ago, a dear friend, Fay Nicholls-Holt, intro-duced me to TAHITIAN NONI® Juice .I began taking it only as a maintenance dose of 1 ounce per day. Shortly afterwards, I noticed a number of areas of health begin to improve. Due to the nature and number of drugs that I have to take daily, passing

urine had become both difficult and painful. The noni juice improved this—not by a huge amount but it was noticeably better. It also lowered the amount of insulin I required each day by about 20 percent.

"The most significant change was in the area of my mind and my general well being. It is kind of hard to put into words, but I wasn't as depressed, and I felt more uplifted as a person. So, the next most obvious thing to do was to increase the dose, which I did from 1 ounce per day to 3 ounces per day. The benefits likewise increased. My urinary problems are much better—about 60 percent gone. My dose of insulin has dropped by about 40 percent. My outlook on life is much more positive. My sickness and the effects of powerful medicines overwhelmed me. Noni juice began to help me get back some control over my life by first, making me feel better, and second opening my mind to looking at things other than conventional medicines. Western medicine is very good, it has saved millions of lives, but it also has many limitations and problems such as bad side effects.

"I thank God for creating noni, which has been the starting point of better health and a better quality of life for my family and me."

Simply put, depression is a mood disorder. We will start this discussion with what someone in David's situation might experience. He may have an adjustment disorder with depression, which can include among other symptoms, a depressed mood. In response to stressor(s)—not including bereavement—one may, as David did, feel very sad, hopeless about his situation, and possibly tearful. Usually within six months, if the stressor is resolved, the person feels back to him or herself. If the stressor is chronic, the depression may last much longer until things get resolved. Examples of such situations could be a long-term disabling illness or the dissolution of a family. Or the response could be in relation to a big life change such as going away from home, moving to a new city, getting a new job or losing a job. Situations like these may take a long time from which to recover and may be very painful to resolve.

Whatever the initial trigger, depression is perhaps one of the most expensive diseases in the United States. According to the National Depressive and Manic Depressive Association, the United States loses an estimated 43 billion dollars a year in missed work-days and less productivity. In addition, there are medical costs from depression's debilitating symptoms, to say nothing of the mental anguish for the patient, his or her family, and friends. Depression affects a person's mood, thoughts, behaviors, and physical well being. As mentioned, it often accompanies or may be sparked by the diagnosis of other chronic illnesses. Statistics show that 80 to 90 percent of all depression cases can be treated very effectively if people would get the mental help they need.[19] The earlier a person gets treatment, the better. It's never too late.

Most depressions are a disorder of the brain's chemistry. However, the disease is much more complex than it sounds. We have already discussed Adjustment Disorder with depression, which appeared to be the case with David. Now to try and understand other kinds of depression better, let's examine three other main categories of depression: major depressive illness, dysthymia, and bipolar disorder.

Major depression strikes intensely for an undetermined period of time, during which time things such as eating, sleeping, or even getting out of bed become almost unbearable. Much of the time one can't think right, or concentrate.

Dysthymia, on the other hand, can be milder and persistent with low moods almost every day, possibly lasting for several years. Sad days outnumber good days. Victims function to a degree, but always feel as if they are never at their full capacity.

Victims of bipolar disorder swing between episodes of major depression and "highs" known as mania or less severe highs, known as hypomania. Its high symptoms include irritability, elevated mood with decreased need for sleep, excessive talking, and impulsive behavior fueled by bad judgment leading to painful consequences for themselves and their loved ones.

Chemicals in the brain may be largely responsible for depression, mania, and hypomania. Serotonin is one such known chemical. Studies on *Morinda citrifolia* reveal an important role it may play in the body's production and proper utilization of serotonin.[20] Noni's ability to modulate other natural biochemicals such as hormones might be why many people have felt less depressed after drinking noni juice. Depression, major depression, dysthymia, and bipolar disorder often require psychiatric help and medicines to normalize the chemicals in the brain.

In my survey, of the 1,512 people who consumed noni juice for help with their depression, 80 percent reported improvement.

Amount of Noni Usage: The average amount consumed by the 80 percent who reported positive results was 3 ounces per day.

Section Seven: Multiple Sclerosis & Parkinson's Disease

Multiple Sclerosis, also known as MS, is a chronic disease of the central nervous system. The disease begins with the destruction of myelin—the fatty sheath that insulates nerve fibers in the central nervous system. Typically, diagnosis of the disease occurs between 20 and 40 years of age. Early symptoms of the condition include difficulty in walking, abnormal sensations such as numbness or pins and needles, eye pain and loss of vision, slurred speech, tremors, and loss of coordination. The natural history of MS is for people to show improvement, get worse, and the cycle repeats. Symptoms become more severe over time, with less improvement in between.

The cause of MS is a very actively researched topic in the medical world. Like many other chronic diseases, genetics appear to play a part in a person's susceptibility to multiple sclerosis. In the United States, the average person has a 1 in 1,000 chance of developing MS. However, those numbers increase to 1 in 100 if a person has close family relations (parents, siblings) already diagnosed with the disease. In addition to genetics, researchers believe viruses, environmental pollutants, and immune system factors may also trigger multiple sclerosis.[21]

Since it is the nervous system that is under attack in those suffering from multiple sclerosis, it is natural to link noni's success in promoting a healthy nervous system with its reported success in relieving some of the negative effects caused by MS. The destruction of the myelin sheath and other affected areas may be helped by noni's ability to rejuvenate "sick" cells throughout the body.

In this same way, noni may also be beneficial to the more than one million Americans who sufferer from Parkinson's disease, another central nervous system disorder that is characterized by uncontrollable movement that grows worse over time. Parkinson's is characterized by low levels of a brain chemical called dopamine. Dopamine, a neurotransmitter, is what transports signals to the brain for movement and coordination. What scientists don't understand is why in Parkinson's patients the brain cells that make dopamine die at a faster rate than normal.

Some symptoms of Parkinson's are:
- impaired balance and coordination
- slow movement
- stiffness of the limbs and trunk
- tremor of the hands, arms, legs, jaw, and face

The risk for Parkinson's disease increases with age. Some scientists have suggested that Parkinson's disease may be caused by toxins that selectively destroy brain neurons connected with the production of dopamine. For example, scientists know of toxins that can cause Parkinson's-like symptoms, such as the toxin MPTP. Typical treatment for people with Parkinson's includes medication, surgery, and physical therapy. Unfortunately, many patients experience negative side effects from the medications such as dry mouth, nausea, dizziness, confusion, hallucinations, drowsiness, and insomnia.

In my survey, of the 25 people who consumed noni juice for help with their symptoms from **multiple sclerosis**, 52 percent reported their symptoms lessened after taking noni juice. The average amount consumed by people with MS was 3.5 ounces per day.

In my survey, of the 25 people who consumed noni juice for help with their symptoms from **Parkinson's disease**, 52 percent reported their symptoms lessened after taking noni juice. The average amount consumed by people with Parkinson's was 3.5 ounces per day.

"She Held Her Head"—*Gale, a sufferer of multiple sclerosis*

Joan L. Mailing, a registered massage therapist in Ontario, Canada, relates the following story:

"My patient Gale was diagnosed with MS in February 1998. Every time she came to me I noticed something different about her walk. I asked her what was wrong with her foot because she was placing it on the floor very gently. She said nothing was wrong with her foot. So I asked her about her leg and thigh—if there was any pain. The answer was no. Later she was diagnosed with multiple sclerosis. Last October I called Gale to tell her about noni. She wanted to get some immediately.

"In December I went to visit her to see how she was doing. I asked her how long it had been since she had an attack. She said three months. One other thing that I had noticed was that Gale had lost weight. Her walk was different and she was not stooped over. Her posture was straighter. She said she lost 10 pounds due to noni juice. Her walk was very even and the strides were wider. Before noni, she was taking steps like a baby and waddling back and forth. The thing I could not get over was her posture. Her spine was straighter and she seemed taller as she held her head up."

Section Eight: High Blood Pressure, Heart Disease, and Stroke

High blood pressure is one of the most noticeable red flags indicating a person's heart and blood vessels are in trouble. Once a person is diagnosed with high blood pressure, he or she is seven times more likely to suffer a stroke, four times more likely to have a heart attack, and five times more likely to die of congestive heart failure. On a positive note, there are well-proven ways to control blood pressure and even reverse some of the damage already done.

Before discussing how to control high blood pressure, let's talk about what it is. Blood pressure is the force exerted by the heart on the blood as it moves through a person's arteries. If a person has high blood pressure, this means the heart is pumping harder than it should have to pump. A healthy blood pressure would read below 120/80, preferably 110/76 or lower. I consider mildly high blood pressure somewhere around 125/85. Most doctors agree that a blood pressure reading of 160/100 or higher is considered dangerous.

I have lumped high blood pressure, heart disease and strokes together, because they are all interrelated in the body's circulatory system. In a heart attack, there is not enough nutrient rich oxygenated blood to nourish the heart muscle cells. As a result, some heart muscle cells die. When enough heart muscle dies, you have a heart attack. It can be sudden, as a result of a cholesterol/calcium/fibrin clot to the coronary artery, or an embolus, which is a clot that breaks away from another part of your body and ends up clogging your coronary arteries. Another scenario would be if your coronary artery goes into spasm, preventing adequate blood flow, or you can have a small unstable plaque released that goes toward the heart and clogs the coronary artery as well as puts it in more spasm. The end result of all these conditions results in not enough nutrient rich oxygenated blood to sustain heart muscle.

In a stroke, or "brain attack" as some lay people call it, the brain tissue is damaged due to lack of blood flow. The lack of blood can be caused by a blood clot in an artery that has decreased in size because of spasms or atherosclerosis. It can also be caused when a brain (cerebral) artery leaks blood as in a leaking or ruptured aneurysm.

There are many lifestyle changes a person with high blood pressure can make to fight against these conditions. A change in diet to reduce red meat and saturated fats, and to add more fiber and fresh fruits and vegetables is a very good start. Sodium intake should be reduced, and of course one ought to get regular exercise.

I believe the reasons for noni's reported success in helping with high blood pressure are multi-faceted. First of all *Morinda citrifolia* contains scopoletin, which has been scientifically proven to dilate blood vessels resulting in lower blood pressure. A second reason that many use noni for high blood pressure is that this fruit juice from Tahiti helps stimulate the body's production of nitric oxide, a chemical which allows the blood vessels to dilate more easily and be more elastic. The third reason, I believe, is through the xeronine system that promotes a healthy cell structure within the circulatory system.

In my survey, of the 1,869 people who consumed noni juice to help with their high blood pressure, 84 percent reported their blood pressure decreased. Of the 2,158 people who took noni to help with their symptoms of heart disease, 76 percent reported lessened symptoms. Last of all, of the 1,806 people who took noni for help with their stroke symptoms, 53 percent reported it helped.

<u>Amount of Noni Usage:</u> The average amount consumed by the 84 percent who reported positive blood pressure results was 3 ounces per day. Those who reported success with stroke and heart disease took on an average 3.5 ounces per day.

"I Will Take Noni for as Long as I Live"—Michael Sossin

"I started to take noni juice in March 1997. My hope was to get my blood pressure under control. I started with 2 ounces per day, one in the morning and one later in the day before dinner. Since then, I changed that to the last thing I do before going to bed at night. Within the first few days, I noticed I had better energy and my hiatal hernia stopped burning. Within the first two or three months, my doctor noticed that my blood pressure was normalizing. He asked me what I was doing differently, and I told him about the noni juice. Being skeptical, he said if I wished to continue with the product that was fine. It was just juice and it should not harm me. This continued for another year with the results of my hypertension staying in the 120 over 80 ranges. My doctor then asked me if I would supply him with a bottle for himself. Which, of course, I did.

"The doctor reported to me that within the first week he had more energy and feeling of well being. I had mentioned to my physician that I wanted to stop my medications. I said I believed noni juice would do as good or better than the medication, and it is a natural food. He said he wanted to monitor me for a while longer. About three months later he said I could start lowering my medications one at a time by decreasing the amount I was taking. The first drug to change was Adalat XL from 60 mg to 30 mg. After monitoring me for another three months, my physician said I

---

could stop Adalat XL entirely although he wanted me back in for a blood pressure check every week for two months. In addition, he sent me for blood tests to see if I could go off my cholesterol pill.

"I will take noni juice for as long as I live. Noni gives me more energy, a feeling of wellness, and is helping me get off the drug medications I have been on since my minor stroke in 1994. I will continue to take a minimum of 2 ounces per day. My health provider also is starting to believe in noni as he has another of his patients getting noni from me. He too is having good results."

Section Nine: HIV and other Immune System Disorders

HIV is an acronym that stands for Human Immunodeficiency Virus. The virus causes just what its name describes—a deficiency in the human immune system. A person can test positive for HIV but not show any symptoms of the deficiency for years. A person who is HIV-positive who had an opportunistic infection (one that would not have developed if HIV had not been present), or who has a helper T-cell blood less than 200 is considered to have Acquired Immunodeficiency Syndrome (AIDS).

There are actually two types of HIV viruses: Type 1, which is more common in the United States, and Type 2, which is more common in Europe. Both may eventually cause AIDS. AIDS becomes life threatening when helper T-cells are weakened or destroyed by the HIV virus. T-cells help infection-fighting antibodies to form in the body's blood. A normal T-cell count is anywhere between 600 and 1,000.

The only way to confirm whether or not a person has the HIV virus or has developed AIDS is to have a blood test. Symptoms of the disease are random and vary from person to person. However, some of the more common signs and symptoms of AIDS can be rapid weight loss, dry cough, recurring fever, night sweats, swollen lymph glands, chronic diarrhea, white spots in the mouth, pneumonia, memory loss, skin lesions, and depression.

Not only have I received reports about how noni has helped reduce the negative signs and symptoms experienced by sufferers of AIDS such as respiratory illnesses and digestive disorders, but I have also received information from individuals indicating that a significant rise in T-cells occurred after starting to drink noni juice. Some believe in the case of noni and AIDS, there may be a very strong relationship between Dr. Ralph Heinicke's work with the xeronine system and boosting the cells most involved with the disease—helper T-cells. In his theory, when the proxeronine is combined with proxeroninease it creates the cell-rejuvenating substance known as xeronine. If the T-cells rejuvenated and present in a larger number, the body should be more able to ward off diseases and maintain functionality.

There are other immune system problems that are not related to HIV. For example, Myasthenia Gravis and Addison's disease are both disorders within the body where the immune system turns against the body. In Myasthenia Gravis, the body creates antibodies against its own nicotinic acetylcholine receptors found in the nerve-muscles synapses. This results in muscular weakness and fatigue.

Addison's disease occurs when the immune system attacks the body's adrenal gland where some of the body's hormones are produced. Without the production of these hormones, the body does not grow correctly, the person will have a chronic, worsening fatigue, blood pressure falls easily, and he or she will be very susceptible to other diseases such as the flu.

With these types of immune system disorders, I believe noni juice can help in several ways. First of all, it can help from a preventative standpoint. If your immune system is not functioning correctly, then a person needs to be very careful about not contracting other common illnesses that could explode into major illness episodes. Noni modulates the overall immune system of the body and helps to maintain optimal health. Many frequent travelers report they drink noni while traveling, when the body's immune defenses seem to be lower. Ancient Polynesian warriors used to take the noni fruit with them to help them maintain stamina and strength when they traveled from island to island

Another way in which noni may help with immune system disorders, according to Dr. Heinicke, is through the cellular rebuilding mechanism referred to as the xeronine system.[22] He believes that the xeronine system may help jump-start the organ or organs that have been attacked by the malfunctioning immune system. The late Dr. Mona Harrison, a Harvard graduate who studied and used TAHITIAN NONI® Juice in her medical practice, theorized that noni plays an important role in stimulating some of the glands of the endocrine system and thereby promotes better hormone production and balance in the body.[23]

In my survey, of the 150 people who consumed noni juice because they were HIV positive, 55 percent reported some sort of beneficial results. Also in my survey, I found that of the 3,707 people who took noni to help with other immune system problems, 77 percent noticed a decrease in their negative symptoms.

<u>Amount of Noni Usage:</u> The average amount consumed by the 55 percent who reported positive results with their HIV symptoms was 3.5 ounces per day. The 77 percent who reported positive results with other immune system problems also drank an average of 3.5 ounces per day.

"The Doctors and Nurses Couldn't Believe It"—Paul Miller, brother to AIDS survivor

"My name is Paul Miller. I am a UPS driver and would like to take this time to share with you a true miracle—one that I wouldn't believe if I hadn't seen it for myself.

"It started Dec. 27, 1998 when I received a phone call from my sister, Deborah Gear, in Port Orange, Florida. She said she needed to talk to me as soon as possible, so I went over that night. She said she was having slurred speech and she was going to Halifax Hospital to run some tests. After two weeks in the hospital and another two weeks waiting for the results, the bad news finally came. My sister, who has been a nurse for 12 years, was diagnosed as HIV-positive and had a condition called PML. PML is a rare form of AIDS and is very deadly. She had about two months to live. In short PML is AIDS of the brain. By the second week of February my sister's right side was completely paralyzed, and her speech was down to saying yes and no. She went down hill very fast from week to week. I prayed to God if there was any answer for her please let me find it. By the week before Easter the spot on her brain covered about 70 percent of its mass. She was totally incoherent, didn't know who I was, her viral load was over 800,000, her T-cell count was under 100 and she had seven sores on her leg that wouldn't heal. She weighed 89 pounds.

"Dr. Hall took her off her HIV medication at that point and put her into a Hospice facility in Port Orange to die. He said she had five days left, ten at best. That was on the Friday before Easter. I was on vacation the next week and I knew I would be going to a funeral.

"Friday before I got off work a friend of mine named Ricky told me about a product that might help her called TAHITIAN NONI® Juice. He told me all about it and then I told him that nothing would help her now, that she was too far gone, but he talked me into buying her a bottle of hope even though I knew it wouldn't help her.

"On Saturday I took it to her and told her all about it, though she didn't know I was there. I told the nurses to start giving it to her 6 to 8 ounces a day. They were reluctant and checked with the doctor. Dr. Hall said she could have it, but it wouldn't help her and the nurses thought the same, but said they would start giving it to her.

"Three days later, while on vacation, I went to see her; she had started reacting to the noni juice. She was somewhat coherent and was trying to say words though you couldn't understand a word. Her Dad, the doctor, and myself thought it was just her last gasp for life before the end. I came back on Saturday only to see more improvement. She was saying yes and no and was a lot more coherent. She had gained six pounds and the sores on her leg appeared to be healing. It seemed too good to be true. It had been a week of improvement but no one believed it could be the juice, but at this time she was only on sleeping pills, painkillers and noni juice. I started to wonder if it was the noni.

"I have seen her every week since. By the second week on noni, her sores were completely healed. She was eating like a horse and was gaining about five pounds a week and was speaking more and more, even in sentences by week three.

"By week four on noni, she started moving her paralyzed leg and a few days later she started moving her arm. Every week she got better and better. The doctors and nurses couldn't believe it. Even though they had a hard time saying it they too came to the conclusion that it was the noni juice. She is now walking and talking though she has a long way to go.

"On June 30 she was released from Hospice and went home. She now weighs 132 pounds, her normal weight. God did let me find the answer; it was a plant that he created that saved her life.

"It is now July 10, 1999, and the new tests are in. Her viral load and her T-cell count are totally normal; her CAT scan showed a decrease of the spot on her brain from 70 percent mass to about 3 percent. The density of the spot that's left is very thin which the doctors say indicates the spot is dissolving itself.

"My sister is no longer dying, though she has a long way to go with physical therapy, speech therapy and time to get back and learn the things she forgot how to do. In time she will be okay. I have my sister back and I thank God and noni juice for that. Noni will change your life forever. It has mine and I'll never forget it."

Section Ten: Acute and Chronic Pain

Pain. We all know what it feels like, but do we know what it really is? When you cut your finger, nerves around the injury send pain signals to the brain, which in return sends impulses back to the injured area that sensitize it and cause inflammation. These signals and impulses last for a relatively short time period and then stop if the pain is acute or relatively brief. However, many researchers believe chronic pain is a different story.

In the book, *The Pain Cure*, Dr. Dharma Khalsa demonstrates how chronic pain may gain a life of its own by in a sense jamming the nervous system pathways and forcing them to stay open. For example, in a painful condition that is chronic, such as back problems, as the pain signals and impulses are sent to and from the brain they begin to engrave a pain pathway on the body's nervous system. Biological "gates" through which pain signals and impulses pass may become jammed open with constant use. Therefore, even after the original injury should have been resolved, the pain continues, becoming an illness, and taking a life of its own.[24]

Things such as lack of sleep, stressful lifestyle, repeated injury, physical inactivity, lack of important dietary nutrients, hypoglycemia, and a serotonin or endorphin deficit may cause the body to jam open its biological gateways and experience chronic pain. Some of the most common types of chronic pain include arthritis, back pain, and migraine headaches.

The ancient native healers, the Kahunas, traditionally used noni for both acute and chronic pain. Many times parts of noni plant and fruit were applied topically to injured areas of the body. Modern science has shown that some of noni's pain-relief agents include terpenes, found in essential oils, which are known to aid in cell synthesis and cell rejuvenation. Other essential nutrients in noni that may work synergistically in pain-relief are proteins, amino acids, enzymes, vitamins and minerals.

In addition, some scientists believe that noni is associated with the body's production of a very important biochemical known as serotonin, which may involve the xeronine system that is believed to promote the body's ability to ward off pain. Serotonin plays a large role in the healthy function of the brain and nerves, the largest players in the pain cycle. Research has shown that serotonin, triggered by the brain, tells the nerves that first pick up pain signals to calm down.

In my study, of the 6,828 people who consumed noni juice to help reduce their pain, 87 percent reported some successful results.

Amount of Noni Usage: The average amount consumed by the 87 percent who reported pain relief was 3 ounces per day.

"In Only Six Days All Was Completely Repaired"—Gwen Kaese

"A little while ago I had a terrible fall on my face. I lost over a pint of blood, cut the top of my head, had a blood bruise on my eye, my nose had a 1/4-inch deep gash across the bridge, and more cuts on my nose and my cheek. I cut my lips on three places on the outside and multiple places on the inside, plus I loosened five teeth. My eye was swollen almost shut, my nose was double in size and my mouth was triple in size all on the left side of my face.

"In only six days all was completely repaired and back to normal except for the cuts on the inside of my mouth! However, my teeth were back strong again!

"I took a Q-tip and put noni juice directly on all cuts inside and out and on all bruises three times a day, washing my face in a splashing motion between each application. (I could not touch my face it was so bad.) I also applied noni oil on top of the noni juice and of course drank extra noni juice. The pain that I experienced was lower.

"My mouth was so swollen and my teeth hurt so much that I couldn't eat. I practically lived on the Morinda protein drinks. My face skipped the black and blue stage and went directly to yellow before it healed. The doctor said if he had not seen it with his own eyes, he would not believed that a 60-year-old woman, or anyone for that matter, could possibly heal with no scabs and be back to normal with new skin in such a short time. He said it was truly a miracle. I was able to be in a family photo scheduled for my birthday six days after the accident."

While the first testimonial dealt with acute pain, here is another example of someone using noni to help relieve symptoms associated with chronic pain.

"My Feet Quit Hurting"—Joanne Ritter

"I take noni juice for the very common fibromyalgia. I have helped others with the same condition. It started back in 1984 when I had to cope with deaths in the family as well as some other problems. I was having my back worked on by a chiropractor, and when he hit the trigger in my back I literally flew up from the table. My treatment was over. Then my feet hurt so badly I could hardly walk. Another doctor worked them out so I could enjoy a trip to Hawaii. I still didn't know until years later why I felt so bad. I would sleep all night and then wake up exhausted. I ached all over like a toothache and popped Advil because I don't take pain easily. All the symptoms matched for fibromyalgia. I took a job where I wouldn't be on my feet all day at an allergy relief product store.

"My boss started distributing noni products. I had never heard of noni, and if someone else had offered me the product I probably would have refused. I was curious about what he was so excited about. My boss said that I would sleep better and have more energy. I didn't notice too much difference until after two bottles. I noticed all my pain was gone and my feet quit hurting. I woke up feeling good. What a difference! My husband thought it was snake oil. He tried noni, and after ten days all the pain from the arthritis in his knees was about gone. He didn't tell me until twelve days later when we had some company from Canada for dinner. He said to them, `I didn't tell Joanne this, but my knees quit hurting two days ago!' I was surprised.

"I got rid of the fibromyalgia symptoms on 1 ounce a day of noni juice, but I take 2 ounces now because it gives me more energy. I up the dose if I get stressed out and start feeling off key. My supply went low at the end of June. I was on 1 ounce a day and my hands got incredibly stiff and painful. In July I went on a super dose for a few days before going back to my regular dose. If I had any doubts as to the effectiveness of noni, I never would have any again. Would I be willing to stay on noni the rest of my life? Of course. I certainly don't want the kind of pain I had back. My husband wouldn't be with out it either."

Section Eleven: Menstrual Disorders

While usually not considered life threatening, severe menstrual disorders can disrupt a woman's life to the point of significant dysfunction. There are many different types of menstrual disorders. In this section I will briefly cover only some of the most common.

It is reported that about three-quarters of all women have uncomfortable physiological and psychological symptoms as they approach menstruation. This condition has been classified as PMS, or premenstrual syndrome, and it ranges from mild to severe. Other menstrual disorders include amenorrhea, which is the absence of menstruation; menorrhagia, or heavy bleeding; and dysmenorrhea, also known as severe menstrual cramps.

Some of the physical symptoms that appear most often during menstruation may not be classified as disorders, but they can cause much discomfort. Bloating, breast tenderness, temporary weight gain, gastrointestinal distress, headaches, rashes, muscle and joint pain, fatigue, gingivitis, heart pounding, hot flashes, hyper-sensitivity to sounds and smells, agitation, and insomnia are a few such symptoms.

The question many doctors are not fully able to answer is why some women experience severe menstrual problems while others seem relatively unaffected. Researchers believe that the bulk of menstrual disorders stem from the fluctuation in hormone levels. This is called estrogen dominance, where estrogen hormones overpower progesterone hormones. In a book I co-authored with Dr. Richard Passwater and Rita Elkins M.H. called Soy Smart Health, we detail how an estrogen and progesterone imbalance may affect women.

Other hormones besides these two have been implicated in menstrual problems. As one example, women who have ovarian cysts have been shown to have higher amounts of androgens, or male hormones, in their systems. The hormone prolactin, when present in high quantities in women who are not pregnant or breast-feeding, can inhibit ovulation-causing amenorrhea. Either too much or too little thyroid hormone can also cause menstrual problems.[25]

If the body were able to maintain more regular hormone levels during menstruation, perhaps many of the signs and symptoms of menstruation could be diverted. This is one area in which I believe noni juice may play an important role.

One of the earliest reported uses of noni by the ancient Kahuna healers was for "women's issues." Little did they know that there is a substance found in noni that was also found in a natural supplement in the 1950s called bromelain. This substance was vigorously researched by large pharmaceutical companies as a treatment for, among other things, severe menstrual cramps. Much of Dr. Ralph Heinicke's work about xeronine came from these original studies on bromelain.

In my survey, of the 3,798 women who consumed noni juice to help reduce painful and uncomfortable menstrual symptoms, 79 percent reported successful results.

Amount of Noni Usage: The average amount consumed by the 79 percent who reported positive results was 2.5 ounces per day.

"I Have No More Abdominal Pain or Mood Swings"—Michelle Titus

"I am a 39-year-old who has had problems with my menstrual cycle since age 12. Each month I would have nausea, diarrhea, lower back pain, burning and severe pain in my abdomen, and headaches. At age 24, I was diagnosed with endometriosis. I also had cysts on my ovaries. After a partial hysterectomy, the doctors assured me the pain and other symptoms were normal each month. Six years later all the symptoms returned.

"My menstrual period has been a living nightmare until January 1999 when I met Jeannette Komsi and she introduced me to noni. Within minutes after taking my first dose, my sinus headache was gone. It was unbelievable. I have no more abdominal pain or mood swings, and my energy level has increased dramatically. I now work six days a week, compared to the four days I used to work. My dose of noni is usually 2 ounces in the morning, but occasionally I increase it to 4 ounces in the evening if I am feeling tension. I plan to take noni forever! When I talked to my physician, he said he didn't know anything about noni but to go ahead and keep taking it, `if you feel better.' You bet I will!"

Section Twelve: Obesity

A startling two-thirds of all adult Americans fall under the National Heart, Lung, and Blood Institute's parameters as being significantly overweight. That means that more than 100 million Americans are at increased risk to develop a myriad of serious health conditions that have been linked to being overweight and obese. Just a few of these conditions include: hypertension, lipid disorders, type 2 diabetes, coronary heart disease, stroke, gallbladder disease, osteoarthritis, sleep apnea, respiratory problems, and even certain cancers. It is no wonder that weight has become much more than just a social issue in the United States. It is one of this nation's major public health challenges. [26]

Most tests for obesity are based on more than just one's weight. Tests usually include information on a person's percentage of body fat, key measurements such as a waist or arm circumference, and a Body Mass Index (BMI). Weight, however, can be an initial indicator of overall health, and it is much easier to access than the body's fat percentage or a BMI.

As seen from the previous sections, noni juice has an array of health boosting ingredients and is reported by many to help the body function on a higher level. Many who suffer from obesity indicate that they experience extreme fatigue doing day-to-day activities, or doing any kind of exercise. However, in my survey 16,056 people out of 25,314 who drank noni juice reported an increase in energy. This increase in energy alone may help those who suffer from being overweight or obese maintain a more active lifestyle that translates into weight loss and better fitness.

Other ways in which noni may help someone loose weight are by promoting better sleep, aiding in the regulation of blood sugar levels (diabetes is closely associated to weight gain), and by boosting the number of antioxidants in the body. For example, we now know that without enough sleep, the body's metabolism may decrease, making it difficult for people to lose weight. Lack of sleep decreases the release of the body's Growth Hormone. GH helps regulate the body's proportion of fat and muscle during adulthood. A reduction in GH also can cause a decrease in metabolism.

In my survey done on noni juice drinkers, I found a large majority of people report they sleep better when drinking noni juice. Of the 2,025 people who consumed noni juice to help improve sleep, 75 percent reported positive results consuming an average of 2.5 ounces per day.

Antioxidants also help people lose weight because they help slow down the aging process as well as restore health on a cellular level. If the body's cells are sick, its survival functions may be to put the body into high gear. Survival functions include holding onto weight for upcoming "hard times," like a bear going into hibernation. If you increase your antioxidants by drinking noni, you may help the body lose weight by increasing cellular health and taking it out of "survival mode."

In my survey, of the 5,526 people who drank noni juice to help with their weight problems, 72 percent reported that they indeed lost weight.

<u>Amount of Noni Usage:</u> The average amount consumed by the 72 percent who reported positive results was 2.5 ounces per day.

"My Recipe for Weight Loss"—Dan Ritchie

"About one month ago I starting drinking homemade shakes containing TAHITIAN NONI® Juice (see recipe below) every one to two days. I have already lost 15 pounds. I know this doesn't sound like a lot of weight, but since I am only about 20 pounds over my ideal weight, I feel great. I can tell that noni is doing what it is suppose to do. The amazing thing to me is that other than the noni shake, I have not changed my diet at all. I still eat meat, pasta, and (dare I say) junk food. I don't work out or exercise anymore than I did before, but I have still lost weight. Honestly the only thing I have changed is that I started the noni juice in the form of a shake."

The shake recipe is as follows:

1 Noni Fiber pack
2 scoops of the Tahiti Trim protein shake
1 – 2 scoops of ice milk or lowfat ice cream
2 ounces of TAHITIAN NONI® Juice

Another noni enthusiast sent this delicious noni bar recipe:

Trudy's Noni Bars

1 C. Tahitian Noni Chocolate Protein Powder
1 C. non-fat dry milk
1/2 C. oatmeal (1 minute)
1/2 C. honey or maple syrup
1/3 C. creamy peanut butter
1/2 C. sesame seeds (optional)
3-4 Tbl. of water

Mix all ingredients together until well blended and smooth. Spray an 8x8 glass or metal pan with cooking spray. Press mixture into pan. Refrigerate 1 hour. Cut into 8 sections. Each section equals one meal. Be sure to drink a large glass of water with your bar.

Approximately per bar there are:
7 grams of fat
33 grams of carbohydrates
10 grams of protein
191 calories
5 grams of fiber

* Credit for this recipe goes to Trudy Crow for creating it and Bonnie Clay for sharing it with me.

Section Thirteen: Kidney Disease

What would your neighborhood look like if the waste disposal system, such as the weekly garbage pickup in front of your house, were canceled for a year? Not a happy thought, right? Now, just take that scenario and relate it to the body. In the body, our kidneys basically serve the function of taking out the trash. The process is done when the blood is circulated through the kidneys. The kidneys remove any waste from the blood and expel it into the urine. Not only do our kidneys remove waste, but also they also extract the important nutrients from the urine and then reabsorb them into the blood stream. When the kidneys fail to work properly, the body becomes sick as its own waste-filled blood slowly poisons its other systems. One such substance is urea, and the basis for uremia. If left untreated, this results in death.

What causes the kidneys to stop working properly? There are actually a large number of related diseases that may cause kidney and urinary tract diseases. I will mention only a few of them in this book. Urologic disease, benign prostatic hyperplasia (BPH), diabetes mellitus (Types 1 and 2), high blood pressure, kidney cancer, and glomerulonephritis all are related to chronic kidney failure. According to the National Kidney Foundation, diabetes and high blood pressure account for 57 percent of all end-stage renal disease.[27] In end-stage renal disease, the patient must engage in a process called dialysis, which acts as an artificial kidney located outside of the body, or obtain a kidney transplant. Dialysis is very expensive, time consuming, and not nearly as efficient as an actual kidney. It may serve, however, to keep the person alive until he or she can obtain a transplant or until his or her kidneys start working again.

Unfortunately surgical transplantation may also have many drawbacks. The body receiving the implant may fail to accept the new kidney, and the fact that there are not enough organs available to all who need new kidneys are just a few of the challenges with transplantation.

The best method, of course, to combat kidney disease is prevention. A lifestyle for healthy people includes drinking at least one quart of water a day, exercise, a healthy diet full of fiber, fruits and vegetables, and using natural supplements. This may not only reduce a person's weight and high blood pressure, but that sort of lifestyle reduces the chance of developing cancer and an assortment of other health conditions.

The following seven items are important warning signs of kidney and urinary tract diseases.[28]

1. Burning or difficulty during urination.
2. More frequent urination, especially at night.
3. Passage of blood appearing in the urine.
4. Puffiness around eyes, swelling of hands and feet, especially in children.
5. Pain in small of back just below the ribs that is not aggravated by movement.
6. High blood pressure.
7. Diabetes (Type I or II).

By incorporating a natural supplement such as noni into an already healthy lifestyle, you may be augmenting your chance to stay clear of many of the diseases that lead to chronic kidney failure. In addition, much research has been done to show that noni has important constituents that boost and sustain cellular integrity. Please refer back to Dr. Mian-Ying Wang's research in Figures 1 and 2 in the cancer section that show the decrease in adduct markers (a test for cancer) in the kidneys of the mice, that were given over time, a mixture containing 10 percent noni juice. Male mice showed a 90% protection, and female mice a 80% protection from developing cancer.

It is good to note that in end-stage renal failure, a patient's food intake is carefully monitored since high levels of potassium can cause a heart attack. TAHITIAN NONI® Juice contains 28.52 milligrams of potassium per ounce. This level is less than half the potassium level found in an ounce of orange juice or tomato juice, as determined by the U.S. Department of Agriculture Nutrient Data Laboratory. Further, grape, pineapple, and apple juices contain higher levels of potassium than TAHITIAN NONI® Juice. The US RDA (United States Recommended Dietary Allowance) for potassium is 2,000 mg per day, seventy times higher than the level found in one ounce of noni juice. However, if you are in end-stage renal failure and have questions as to whether the level of potassium in noni juice would be a problem, I suggest following the advice of your physician.

In my survey, of the 3,764 people who consumed noni juice in order to augment their kidneys' health, 67 percent reported successful results.

Amount of Noni Usage: The average amount consumed by the 66 percent who reported positive results was 2 ounces per day.

"What a Gift to Mankind"—Cliff Blumberg

"My ordeal started with feeling terrible and running a fever of 101. My internist misdiagnosed this as the flu. I had no other symptoms that suggested the flu. I just didn't feel right! After one week of being away from my dental practice, I developed soreness in my groin, which prompted me to go to the emergency room of

the North Shore hospital where x-rays and a CAT scan and urine analysis revealed a kidney stone. This was confirmed the following day with IVP x-rays.

"While in the emergency room I was surrounded by two patients in severe, climbing-the-wall pain. They too were passing kidney stones. Both were on morphine and the pain was still excruciating. I had no pain. During this entire two-week period from initial onset to actually passing the stone, I increased my consumption of TAHITIAN NONI® Juice from my usual 3 ounces every morning to an additional 3 ounces during the day. At no time did I have the usual severe pain associated with passing of a kidney stone. Just another confirming personal experience that noni juice works! What a gift to mankind!"

Section Fourteen: Skin and Hair Problems

Our skin and hair has to last a lifetime. The care that you take now will make a difference on how you look as you get older. The development of gray hair, facial wrinkles, and changes in skin coloration and texture represent the aging process. And with aging comes the loss of elasticity and decreased collagen. However, according to Dr. Scott Gerson, M.D., environmental factors cause many of these changes, especially unprotected exposure to sun, wind, heat, chemical preservatives, and radiation.[29] In addition there are many other skin problems that can affect the young people, such as skin discoloration, non-cancerous growths, as well as other conditions. The good news, whether you are young or old, is that many skin and hair conditions are preventable and even reversible.

In many cases, helping your skin is based on increasing a connective tissue component involved in skin and hair called *collagen*. Whether you have dry, rough skin or dry, brittle hair, there are ways to naturally build up your collagen levels and restore needed nutrients to your hair and skin.

Hair is an appendage of the skin, so if something is applied to the hair it also applied to the skin and vice versa. Trauma from environmental factors is one of the major culprits of hair, scalp, and skin injury. When used both internally and topically, noni juice has several ingredients that have been scientifically proven beneficial for the body's skin, such as three essential polyunsaturated fatty acids: linoleic, linolenic, and arachidonic. Essential polyunsaturated fatty acids cannot be manufactured by the body; they must be ingested as a food supplement. These acids help counteract hair, scalp and skin trauma, as well as, prevent dryness, and maintain its integrity.

Noni juice also contains glycerol, fatty acids, and butyric acids, all which also fight against excessively dry, rough skin. In addition, noni contains caprylic and capric acids that combine with glycerol to produce triglycerides. These triglycerides lubricate the skin, scalp, and hair. They work in concert with the other nutrients in noni to help maintain skin and hair smoothness, plumpness, and luster.

In my survey, of the 877 people who used noni juice in order to enhance their skin or hair, 78 percent reported successful results.

<u>Amount of Noni Usage:</u> The average amount used by the 78 percent who reported positive results with their skin and hair was 2 ounces per day.

"We Gave Him an Ounce a Day"—Doug Alcorn, Grandfather

"In January 2001 it was discovered that my grandson Dillon had a polyp growing in his nose. The family doctor said he would schedule surgery for Dillon as soon as possible. In April, we discovered noni and, with still no word from the doctor, we decided to try it on Dillon.

"By this time the polyp had grown to completely block off his nostril and was protruding from his nose a bit. The kids at school were teasing him about it now and I could see a fight coming. He is only 9 years old, but big for his age. We gave him an ounce a day and dabbed some noni directly on the polyp at bedtime. In ten days the polyp was completely gone! We didn't say anything to the doctor about this at the time, as we were curious to see how long it might take to have surgery scheduled.

"It was August before we got the call from the doctor's office saying that surgery had been scheduled. That left us wondering what the polyp might have looked like by this time if we hadn't used the noni. Well, a few months later, we had our answer when we spotted a gentleman crossing the street in busy downtown traffic. His polyp was down to his chin and was as big as a golf ball! We felt let down by the medical services here, and are thankful for those who have brought noni to the world."

Section Fifteen: Smoking

Cigarette smoking is an addiction that is related to more than 400,000 deaths in the United States each year. In fact, statistics show that every cigarette you smoke shortens your life by 14 minutes. If you smoke, you increase your risk for lung cancer, emphysema, coronary heart disease, and the list goes on and on. Sadly, not only does smoking harm the smoker, but it can also harm family members, coworkers, and friends through secondhand smoke. In babies up to age 18 months, secondhand smoke is related to approximately 300,000 cases of bronchitis and pneumonia each year. Second hand smoke also increases a child's risk for contracting middle ear problems, coughing, wheezing, and asthma.

So many smokers want to quit smoking but have a hard time both physically and emotionally because of the nicotine addiction that smoking causes. To quit smoking, you may find it best to instigate some behavioral changes as well as trying a natural supplement such as noni.

It was during Dr. Heinicke's research on bromelain when he discovered a possible link between breaking addictions and xeronine. He ran several small, informal experiments to see if by increasing a person's intake of proxeronine and xeronine, someone could quit smoking more easily. His results were extremely positive. Addictions specialist Dr. William McPhilamy has also had a lot of success using noni in his medical practice.

In my survey, of the 876 people who consumed noni juice to help them stop smoking, 56 percent reported successful results. That is, they stopped smoking for one month or longer.

<u>Amount of Noni Usage:</u> The average amount consumed by the 56 percent who reported positive results with smoking was 3 ounces per day. The majority of the noni users who stopped smoking swished 1 ounce of noni juice around in their mouth for five minutes before swallowing it just before breakfast, lunch, and dinner.

"I Was Not Craving Cigarettes"—Sheri Zahler, 33-year-old mother

I was nine years old when I started smoking. Each time I tried to quit the cravings for cigarettes would come back, especially when I had extra stress. In January of 2000, my mother gave me a bottle of TAHITIAN NONI® Juice. Initially, I didn't start taking noni to stop smoking. I took it just because my mom said it would make me feel better. At first I took it a bit sporadically. I would be really good for a week or two and then forget for a few days. After about one or two months of being on the juice, I realized that I was not craving cigarettes. I then completely stopped smoking—cold turkey. After finally quitting, using the noni juice, the stress level in my life seemed to soar. I had job changes and some relationship difficulties, yet through it all I didn't panic. My mom, who originally introduced me to noni juice, has also stopped smoking."

Section Sixteen: Mental Acuity (Memory and Concentration Difficulties)

In today's world, more people than ever have memory problems. Memory problems before the age of 70 or 80 years of age could be a sign of disease. Severe memory loss can be a sign of dementia, or in other words the loss of former intellectual abilities. The most common form of dementia is Alzheimer's disease.

Alzheimer's disease is named after Dr. Alois Alzheimer, a German doctor. In 1906, Dr. Alzheimer noticed abnormalities in the brain tissue of a woman who had died of an unusual mental illness. In this woman's brain, he found abnormal clumps (amyloid plaques) and tangled bundles of fibers (neurofibrillary tangles), both of which are now known to be symptoms of Alzheimer's.

Each year, Alzheimer's disease affects an increasingly larger percentage of the world's population 65 and older. In fact, the number of individuals diagnosed with Alzheimer's is doubling every five years. The current annual cost is estimated to be in excess of $60 billion dollars. Alzheimer's disease starts slowly and has a specific pattern it follows. Those people with Alzheimer's literally forget routines and habits they have known forever.

While scientists still do not know the exact cause of Alzheimer's, or general dementia for that matter, there are risk factors. Age, family history, high blood pressure, high cholesterol, and low levels of the vitamin folate may predispose people to contracting Alzheimer's. Social isolation is another possible cause of cognitive decline. Environmental toxins and previous brain trauma may also predict the occurrence of Alzheimer's disease.

In addition to Alzheimer's disease, there are other reasons for memory difficulty. Different types of medication (i.e. anti-depressants) for the elderly can cause memory problems as well as a loss of certain nutrients or vitamins such as Vitamin B. Thyroid problems can also impact memory.

Another recent discovery connected to Alzheimer's is that it is associated to inflammation of the brain cells. This inflammation is believed to be caused by the COX 2 enzyme, the same enzyme that is connected to arthritis and some genetic cancers. Noni juice is a proven COX 2 inhibitor, and it may help those with Alzheimer's in this area.

Concentration problems in children (and adults) are another area in which noni has been shown to possibly help. Attention Deficit/Hyperactivity Disorder (ADHD) is a type of neurological illness that affects behavior, mood, and learning. Because it is an illness that is being diagnosed in an overwhelming large number of children, this disorder is seeing a lot of attention as of late. Symptoms of ADHD are inattention, hyperactivity, and impulsive behavior. Please note that some children have the disorder without hyperactivity. Experts say about one child in every classroom has ADHD. Causes are, once again, not certain. However, there does seem to be brain chemistry irregularities in children with ADHD, and the disorder tends to run in families.[30]

In the case of ADHD, noni may be helpful through is ability to modulate the production of the some of the chemicals in the brain, (such as serotonin) as well as increase overall cellular health in the brain.

In my survey, of the 5,543 people who consumed noni juice to help with mental acuity, 73 percent reported successful results.

<u>Amount of Noni Usage:</u> The average amount consumed by the 73 percent who reported positive results with mental acuity was 2 ounces per day.

"All His Grades Started to Improve"—Sherri and Zachary Lipps

"In September of 1998, my eight-year-old son, Zachary, was diagnosed with neurofibromatosis. This disease causes tumors to grow in the nerves and bones throughout his body. Most of this occurs when he hits puberty. We had to see a specialist that was 500 miles away. He told us that with this disease we needed to watch for Attention Deficit Disorder. We were to have a conference with his teachers; they were the important link to watching for changes in his schoolwork, concentration and overall behavior where ADD or ADHD symptoms might start showing up. We were warned that this could also change drastically to fall into mental retardation.

"In November of 1998 my girlfriend, Kristie Knorr, who knew about his condition, introduced me to TAHITIAN NONI® Juice. A life changing experience was about to happen. I started giving Zachary 1 ounce of juice every morning. I also started drinking the juice to support him. I noticed changes in me immediately.

"I have suffered from migraines for 20 years, a migraine every week to two weeks. Because I was drinking noni, the migraines went away, I was so excited! When Zachary got his second quarter report card form school, all his grades started to improve. His

---

C grades turned into B grades, and his B grades turned into A grades. He also moved to the top reading group in his class. I couldn't believe it. His concentration at homework time was unbelievable. We didn't argue every day like we always did in the past. He'd sit down everyday, without complaining, and do his homework. This was a very big improvement for us, very different from the constant arguing for two hours each day. We just got his fourth quarter report card, Zachary received only one B and the rest were A grades! I couldn't believe it. We were so proud of him.

"The only thing that we were doing differently was drinking noni juice. We love this juice. It has changed our lives and has given us a positive outlook on Zachary's future. They have not come up with a cure for this disease yet, but we have found hope through noni juice that Zachary can live with this disease without any major problems. Thank you noni juice for changing our lives."

Section Seventeen: Health Enhancers— Muscle Building, Sexual Enhancement, Better Digestion, Well-being

Due to its cellular enhancing abilities, noni juice is not only helpful to those who suffer from illnesses, but people in already good health also reap its benefits. Some of these health-enhancing benefits I tracked in my survey were muscle building, sexual enhancement, better digestion, and overall well-being. Noni's effectiveness with these conditions may the result of a combination of increased antioxidants, xeronine, and the many phytochemicals found within the natural juice. I have received comments from thousands of people who simply say noni makes them feel better. The following are just two such comments: 42-year-old Dennis Jefferson, who stopped smoking while drinking noni, says, "I love the way it makes me feel." Derrick Bowers, 32, says, "I needed more get up and go. I needed more energy to make it through the day. Now that I drink noni while I'm at work, I'm not tired and my days start out energized."

Of the 1,216 people who consumed noni juice to help increase muscle, 70 percent reported successful results consuming an average of 2 ounces per day.

Of the 2,984 people who consumed noni juice to help improve sexual enhancement, 84 percent reported successful results consuming an average of 2 ounces per day.

Of the 3,171 people who consumed noni juice to help with their digestion, 90 percent reported successful results consuming an average of 2.5 ounces per day.

Of the 7,879 people who consumed noni juice to help with their overall well being, 80 percent reported successful results consuming an average of 2 ounces per day.

"I Felt Better in my Body"— Mika Myllylä, Finland's most accomplished cross-country skier. His Olympic Medals include: 1 Gold, 1 Silver, and 2 Bronze from the Lillehammer 1994 and Nagano 1998 Winter Olympics

"My friend introduced me to TAHITIAN NONI® Juice. He said, 'I give you this bottle. Taste it. Try it. Tell me afterwards what you feel.' When I used it for two weeks I felt better in my body. It is going to be a very important part of my training and nutritional program. It's always with me; I feel a little bit empty when I'm without it."

"I Can Now Eat Almost All Foods"—Dr. Brent Frame, a doctor with digestion difficulties

"I am a board certified foot and ankle surgeon, residency director, and scientific chairman of the New Mexico Podiatric Medical Association. I have had ulcerative colitis for six years. Nothing has helped me very much, except for some severe diet restrictions that helped a little. When my friends Dave and Paula Castle tried to get me to try noni juice in January 1999, I declined, thinking they were just trying to sell me something. I was very stubborn. Six months late my wife brought home a case of juice and said, 'It's paid for. I'm going to try it. You might as well try it too.' So I did. Very skeptically, I started on a loading dose of 2 ounces in the morning and 2 ounces in the evening. (I still drink the same amount today!) I was extremely surprised that within three weeks I felt dramatically better. My colitis was significantly improved within a month. No more running to the toilet 10-12 times a day. For the first time in six years I was totally regular and without any pain."

Question and Answer Section

I receive questions regularly from people who are interested in noni juice and my research, but who don't have a lot of time to study it own their own. The following questions and answers are to serve as a quick reference to those looking for more information about noni juice and my involvement with it.

Q: *Dr. Solomon, how did you get involved with noni?*

A: In 1996, Dr. Richard Passwater, a noted nutritional expert, and I were asked by a publisher of a health journal if we thought it would be worthwhile to do an in-depth article about noni. I had not heard of noni at that time. In the following years, that assignment has taken me around the world to collect data and field studies of literally thousands of scientists, physicians, other health professionals, and noni drinkers. From this material I have written books and articles, made audiotapes, and lectured about noni.

Q: *How many health professionals and noni drinkers did you contact?*

A: I received information from 1,227 Health professionals, representing 25,314 noni juice drinkers.

Q: *You received survey data about noni from how many different countries?*

A: Eighty countries or territories.

Q: *In your travels researching noni, what scientist has made the greatest contribution to understanding the Xeronine System theory?*

A: Dr. Ralph Heinicke, the man who conceived the Xeronine System, has been researching it for over 50 years.

Q: *Are the 29 health conditions you discuss in this book the only documented conditions that noni has been reported to help?*

A: No. There are more studies and research that I have not been able to include in this book because of space limitations. I have many more testimonials from people concerning ailments that I have not mentioned in this book. Since noni has been used for many centuries in French Polynesia as a natural healer, there are many "unscientific" reported uses for all parts of the Morinda citrifolia plant that may still be researched by other scientists.

Q: *Is it true there are published reports that noni made some people sick?*

A: Yes and No. I tracked some of these reports down and found that it was not the noni that made the people ill, but the contaminants, toxins, and impurities inside the noni product. There was not adequate quality control. This is why I try to limit my studies to TAHITIAN NONI® Juice since its manufacturer has unsurpassed quality control. TAHITIAN NONI® Juice is grown and harvested in the pristine environment of Polynesia and is routinely tested for over 300 contaminants by two independent laboratories. Contaminants, toxins, and impurities have not been found in TAHITIAN NONI® Juice.

Q: *Is TAHITIAN NONI® Juice safe for everyone to drink noni juice?*

A: Noni juice comes from a natural food that has been reported to be safe. It has been used by thousands of people worldwide for thousands of years. I have not seen any documented negative reports of using TAHITIAN NONI® Juice for even pregnant and lactating women, children, and the elderly. A few people have reported allergies, hypersensitivities, and other minor problems. As repeated earlier, check first with your health professional. For those people who must carefully watch their potassium intake, TAHITIAN NONI® Juice has less than half the potassium level found in one ounce of orange juice or tomato juice, as documented by the U.S. Department of Agriculture Nutrient Data Laboratory.

Q: ***How does noni help with so many different health conditions?***

A: This is a complex answer. Many of noni's wide-ranging health benefits have been attributed to its ability to boost nitric oxide, as well as for noni's ingredients such as scopoletin, antioxidants, proxeronine, and others. Please refer to my book The Noni Solution for more information.

Q: ***Are there any side effects from taking noni juice?***

A: For nearly all the people who drink noni juice, even in extremely large quantities, there are few, if any, who experience side effects. Less than 1 percent of people are allergic to noni juice. These people may experience a rash, itching, diarrhea, and very occasionally trouble with breathing. Within 24 hours after discontinuing noni, most allergic side effects disappear. Non-allergic side effects are experienced by less than 2 percent of those who drink noni. These people may have slight belching, mild diarrhea, gas, or nausea. These side effects usually decrease or stop within 24 hours after the serving size of noni juice is stopped or decreased by about half of the original amount.

Q: *How much noni should I drink?*

A: The answer to that question is what sparked me to write this book. There is a general guideline found in the section "Amazing Noni Juice" In addition, Table 5 indicates the average amount of noni juice people took who received help with their suffering from 29 different conditions. Table 3 also contains what I call a suggested noni usage amount based on age, weight, and current health status. Using these guidelines, I suggest that you monitor for yourself how much noni you need to achieve the desired effect.

Q: For how long should I drink noni juice?

A: That is up to you. We all have varying needs. My survey showed that 95 percent of those who reported noni was helpful experienced results within three months of starting noni. Therefore, I would give noni at least a three-month trial. Most people who did not obtain optimal results either consumed too little noni juice or didn't take it for a long enough time. For many people, noni is a supplement that they wish to continue drinking for maintenance and preventative purposes all their life. Results from my study showed that 69 percent of those who experienced positive results after drinking noni juice said they would never stop drinking it.

Q: *What is the Commission of the European Communities, and what is its connection to noni as a novel food?*

A: After years of testing and researching, the Commission of the European Communities (much like the FDA in the United States) authorized the sale of TAHITIAN NONI® Juice in Europe as a novel food. The Committee concluded, "There were no indications of adverse effects…on subacute and subchronic toxicity, genotoxicity and allergenicity." TAHITIAN NONI® Juice is the first noni juice product approved for sale in Europe.

Q: *Was TAHITIAN NONI® International recently presented with an award?*

A: Yes, The International Council for Caring Communities (ICCC) presented the "Corporation with Social Responsibility" Award to TAHITIAN NONI® International at the United Nations Headquarters in New York. It was awarded at the "Public-Private Partnership" Luncheon held during the annual "Caring Communities for the 21st Century: Imaging the Possible" International Conference on February 11, 2004.

Q: *Who helped you most in appreciating noni?*

A: A higher power.

ENDNOTES

[1] Solomon, Neil. Happy & Healthy Pets. Orem, Utah: Direct Source, 2003.

[2] Hirazumi, Anne. "Antitumor Studies of a Traditional Hawaiin Medicianl Plant, Morinda citrifolia (Noni), In Vitra and In Vivo." Doctoral dissertation, University of Hawaii: 1997.

[3] 1998 Novel Prize winners: Drs. Robert Fuchgott, Feried Murad, and Louis Igano, Stockholm, Sweden.

[4] 1999 Nobel Prize winner: Guenther Blobel, Stockholm, Sweden.

[5] Solomon, Neil and Cord Udall. The Noni Phenomenon: Discover the Powerful Tropical Healer that Fights Cancer, Lowers High Blood Pressure and Relieves Chronic Pain. Vineyard, Utah: Direct Source Publishing, 1999.

[6] Ibid.

[7] Heinicke, Ralph. The Xeronine System: A New Cellular Mechanism that Explains the Health Promoting Action of Noni and Bromelain. Orem, Utah: Direct Source Publishing, 2001.

[8] M.Y. Wang, W. Bender, and L.F. Yu. "Preventive Effects of Tahitian Noni Juice on the Formation of 7, 12-demethylbenz(a)anthracene (DMBA) DNA Adducts in vivo." Submitted to The Merican Association for Clinical Research, AACR 91st Annual Meeting: April 1-4, 2000, San Francisco.

[9] Hiramatsu, Tomonori and Masaya Imoto, Takashi Koyano, Kasuo Umezawa. "Introduction of Normal Phenotypes in Ras-Transormed Cells by Damnacanthal from Morinda citrifolia," Cancer Letters, Vol. 73, 1993.

[10] M.Y. Wang, W. Bender, and L.F. Yu. "Preventive Effects of Tahitian Noni Juice on the Formation of 7, 12-demethylbenz(a)anthracene (DMBA) DNA Adducts in vivo." Submitted to The Merican Association for Clinical Research, AACR 91st Annual Meeting: April 1-4, 2000, San Francisco.

[11] Wang, M.Y. and C. Su. "Cancer Prevention: Molecular Mechanisms to Clinical Applications," Vol. 952, 161-168. Annals of the New York Academy of Sciences, Dec. 2001.

[12] Solomon, Neil. The Pain Fighter: TAHITIAN NONI" Juice. Orem, Utah: Direct Source Publishing, 2001.

[13] Young, Chafique, and Alain Roland, Jacques Fleurentin, Marie-Clarie Lanhers, Rene Misslin, Francois Mortier, "Analgesic and Behavioural Effects of Morinda citrifolia," Planta Med., Vol. 56, 1990.

[14] Joseph, Jennifer. "Physical Proof of Chronic Pain." http:///abcnews.go.com/sections/living/Daily News/fibromyalgia980408.html.

15 Solomon, Neil and Cord Udall. The Noni Phenomenon: Discover the Powerful Tropical Healer that Fights Cancer, Lowers High Blood Pressure and Relieves Chronic Pain. Vineyard, Utah: Direct Source Publishing, 1999.

16 Carpenter, C.C.J. and N. Solomon, S.G. Silverberg, T. Bledsoe, R.C. Northcutt, J.R. Klinenberg, I.L. Bennett, and A.M. Harvey. 'Schmidt's Syndrome (Thyroid and Adrenal Insufficiency): A Review of the Literature and a Report of Fifteen New Cases, Including Ten Instances of Co-extstent Diabetes Mellitus," Medicine, 1964, 43:153.

17 Solomon, N. and C.C. Carpenter, I.L. Bennett and A.M. Harvey. "Schmidt's Syndrome (Thyroid and Adrenal Inufficiency) and Co-existence of Diabetes Mellitus," Diabetes 14 (1965):300.

18 Well-Connected. "What is Asthma in Adults," http://webmd.lycos.com/content/dmk/dmk_artaicle_5461904.

19 Nordenberg, Liora. "Dealing with the Depths of Depression" http://webmd.lycos.com/content/dmk/dmk_article_1460967.

20 Solomon, Neil and Cord Udall. The Noni Phenomenon: Discover the Powerful Tropical Healer that Fights Cancer, Lowers High Blood Pressure and Relieves Chronic Pain. Vineyard, Utah: Direct Source Publishing, 1999.

21 "MS Information:What are the Symptoms?" http://www.nmss.org./msinfo/symptoms.html.

22 Heinicke, Ralph. The Xeronine System: A New Cellular Mechanism that Explains the Health Promoting Action of Noni and Bromelain. Orem, Utah: Direct Source Publishing, 2001.

23 Harrsion, Mona, M.D. What Else Every Doctor Should Know. Orem, Utah: Direct Source Publishing, 2002.

24 Khalsa, Kharma Singh. The Pain Cure. New York: Warner Book, 1999: 4-10.

25 Solomon, N., and R. Paswater, R. Elkins. Soy Smart Health, Woodland Publishing: Pleasant Grove, Utah, 2000.

26 The National Heart, Lung, and Blood Institute. "First Federal Obesity Clinical Guidelines Released,' http://webmd.lycos.com/content/dmk/dmk_article_58868.

27 National Kidney Foundation. "End Stage Renal Disease in the United States," wysiwyg;//16/http://www.kidney.org/general/news/esrd.cfm.

28 ibid.

29 Gerson, Scott. Noni, Healing, and You. Orem, Utah: Direct Source Publishing, 2001.

30 The National Institute of Mental Health and the American Academy of Pediatrics.